The Fertility Transition in Iran:
Revolution and Reproduction

Mohammad Jalal Abbasi-Shavazi
Peter McDonald · Meimanat Hosseini-Chavoshi

The Fertility Transition in Iran: Revolution and Reproduction

Springer

Mohammad Jalal Abbasi-Shavazi
Department of Demography
Faculty of Social Sciences
University of Tehran
Tehran Iran
mabbasi@ut.ac.ir

Peter McDonald
Australian Demographic
and Social Research Institute (ADSRI)
Australian National University
Canberra
Australia
peter.mcdonald@anu.edu.au

Meimanat Hosseini-Chavoshi
Department of Family Health & Population
Ministry of Health and Medical Education
Hafez Avenue Tehran
Iran
Meimanat.Hosseini@anu.edu.au

ISBN 978-90-481-3197-6 e-ISBN 978-90-481-3198-3
DOI 10.1007/978-90-481-3198-3
Springer Dordrecht Heidelberg London New York

Library of Congress Control Number: 2009930526

Printed on acid-free paper

Springer is part of Springer Science+Business Media (www.springer.com)

Preface

Confounding all conventional wisdom, the fertility rate in the Islamic Republic of Iran fell from 7 births per woman in 1979 to 1.9 births per woman in 2006. That this, the largest and fastest fall in fertility ever recorded, should have occurred in one of the world's few Islamic Republics demands explanation. This is the purpose of this book.

Conventional wisdom has been that falls in fertility in developing countries are gained slowly and only in open societies, particularly those open to the western notion that rapid population growth is an obstacle to economic development. The 'western package' of development, promoted by organizations such as the World Bank and the International Monetary Fund, combines economic reforms including abolition of tariffs, removal of currency controls, private foreign investment, transfer of technology and human capital enhancement with aggressive, government-sponsored family planning programs. Japan provided the first apparent evidence of the appropriateness of this development model and it was followed by other Asian success stories such as South Korea, Singapore, Thailand, and Indonesia. The Islamic Revolution ensured that this 'western package' was not implemented in Iran yet fertility has fallen just as fast if not faster than in those countries where the package was applied. In this book, we address how this occurred.

Various questions have been raised regarding the Iranian fertility transition. What are the reasons for the fall of fertility in Iran? What are the processes through which fertility has fallen? What is the relative importance of social, economic and cultural influences and what has been the role of the family planning program? What are the reasons for the similarity of fertility trends across provinces and in both urban and rural areas? What is the future of fertility in Iran? Will it continue to decline or will it rise again in the future? All these questions are addressed in this book.

We use various datasets including the 1986, 1996 and 2006 Censuses and the 2000 Iran Demographic and Health Survey (IDHS) to examine fertility trends over the last three decades. However, the main findings in the book are drawn from the 2002 Iran Fertility Transition Survey (IFTS) and the 2005 Iran Low Fertility Survey (ILFS) which were specifically designed and implemented to examine socio-economic and cultural determinants of fertility and the dynamics of contraception in Iran.

The book is divided into ten chapters. The first chapter presents the theoretical framework for analysing fertility decline in Iran. The second chapter discusses pre- and post-revolutionary population policies in Iran, and sets out the context within which the fertility decline has occurred. Chapter 3 presents the broad evidence of fertility trends and patterns in Iran up to 2006. Chapter 4 provides a more detailed analysis of fertility trends using parity progression ratios. Chapter 5 deals with marriage change as one of the main proximate determinates of fertility, and examines the extent to which transformation of marriage has contributed to the fertility decline in Iran. Chapter 6 focuses on the trends, levels and patterns of contraceptive use across time, while Chapter 7 uses the unique dataset from the ILFS on the full history of women's contraceptive use, and provides important insights into the changing contraceptive behaviour of successive generations of Iranian married women. This chapter provides a parallel to Chapter 4 that examines the birth histories of women across their lifetimes. Chapter 8 provides a cohort perspective on changes in attitudes related to family and fertility behaviour. The chapter discusses to what extent transformation of attitudes toward family and fertility paved the way for the later success of the family planning program and the phenomenal fertility decline in Iran in recent decades. One of the main features of social change in post-revolutionary Iran is the improvement of women's status within an Iranian–Islamic context. Addressing questions arising from the theories of gender equity and women's autonomy, Chapter 9 discusses how and to what extent the improvement of the status of women in Iran has been linked with contraceptive use and fertility decline. The final chapter reviews the applicability to the Iranian case of the various theories that have been developed to explain the fertility transition, and presents our expectations for the future of fertility in Iran.

This is a comprehensive book and is based on a decade of research collaborations by the authors. It applies theories and hypotheses of fertility decline in explaining the sharpest fall of fertility ever recorded. The book is also rich in data as well as the application of different demographic methods to interpret the data. It offers guidelines for the future of fertility in Iran. We recommend the book to not only demographers and social scientists (sociologists, anthropologists and economists), but also to those who are interested in social and demographic changes in Iran and other Islamic countries in the Middle East. It is also a useful reference for demography students and researchers who are interested in applying fertility theories in designing surveys and analysing data. Finally, the book would be of interest to policy makers who are interested in the past and future of demographic transition in Iran.

Tehran and Canberra
May 2009

Mohammad Jalal Abbasi-Shavazi
Peter McDonald
Meimanat Hosseini-Chavoshi

Acknowledgements

This book is a product of a fruitful collaboration by the authors for a decade. We are indebted to many institutions, universities, and individuals whose contribution, support and comments have been instrumental for the completion of this book.

The Department of Demography of the Faculty of Social Sciences along with Division of Population Research of the Institute for Social Studies and Research of the University of Tehran and the Demography and Sociology Program (now the Australian Demographic and Social Research Institute – ADSRI) of the Australian National University have been the main institutions where the collaborations between the three authors have taken place. The authors met frequently in Tehran and Canberra and benefited from the stimulating and scientific environment at the two universities. We would have not been able to complete the manuscript of this book without the generous institutional support of the two universities. We owe special thanks to our colleagues and graduate students at the Department of Demography of the University of Tehran and the Australian Demographic and Social Research Institute at the Australian National University for their support over the years.

This book is based on the findings of three Wellcome Trust (WT) funded projects which have been implemented since 1998. The first one was a 2 year Postdoctoral Fellowship to the first author during 1998–2000. In this project, fertility trends and patterns in Iran during 1972 and 1996 were analyzed. Several questions arose from this study which led to two further WT funded projects awarded to McDonald and Abbasi-Shavazi. The Iran Fertility Transition Survey (IFTS) was conducted in four provinces of Gilan, West Azarbaijan, Sistan and Baluchistan, and Yazd during 2002–2004. This was followed by another project entitled the Iran Low Fertility Survey (ILFS) which was conducted in the provinces of Yazd, Gilan, Isfahan and the city of Tehran during 2004–2007. We would like to acknowledge the generous support of the Welcome Trust that enabled us to successfully implement the three projects.

We owe many thanks to those who made contributions to the implementation of the IFTS and ILFS surveys. We appreciate the support of Dr Bahram Delavar, the former Director General of the Family Health and Population Department and his colleagues who made the completion of the projects possible. We are also indebted to the Iran Ministry of Health and Medical Education for providing a scholarship to Dr Meimanat Hosseini-Chavoshi, the third author, to complete her Ph.D. in Demography at the ANU. Through this collaboration, Dr Hosseini made a substantial and valuable contribution in the implementation, data collection and analysis of these two projects. Her Ph.D. thesis was based on the findings of these two surveys and three chapters of this book are drawn from her work. We would like to thank the Medical Sciences Universities of Yazd, Rasht, Zahedan, Isfahan, Tehran, Iran, Shahid Beheshti, and Oroumiyeh for their support and involvement in the accomplishment of our two surveys. Our appreciations go to our provincial coordinators, Dr/s Mohammad Abbasi, Foroozandeh Kalantari, Siamak Aghlmand, Ghadirollah Najafizadeh, Soosan Mahmoudi, Sheerin Nasirzad, Shahla Ghanbari and Pejman Aghdak, and also to our interviewers and supervisors whose efforts were valuable in data collection for these projects. The Statistical Center of Iran (SCI) also provided the necessary data from the 1986, 1996, and 2006 censuses. Assistance from Ali Reza Zahedian, Taha Nourollahi, and Neamat Mirfallah Nassiri from the SCI are gratefully acknowledged.

We are also indebted to many colleagues for their valuables comments and questions throughout our projects. The list is long but we would like to name Terence H. Hull, Gigi Santow, Ann Evans, Mohammad Mirzaie, Diana Glazebrook, John C. Caldwell, Arland Thornton, John Casterline, Amir Houshang Mehryar, Zhongwei Zhao, Chris Wilson, Geoffrey McNicoll, Albert Hermalin and the late Ronald Freedman. Gavin Jones and S. Philip Morgan have not only provided useful comments on our earlier papers and research findings, but also thoroughly reviewed the manuscript of this book and provided valuable suggestions for the final version of the book. Several papers have been published based on our surveys as ANU Demography Working Papers, journal articles, book chapters and conference presentations. Several workshops also were held in Tehran to disseminate the results of our surveys. We have benefitted from valuable comments received from participants and anonymous reviewers for each of these publications and presentations.

Many people provided administrative and institutional support for the implementation of the projects and dissemination of the findings of our surveys of whom we would like to acknowledge the support from Taghi Azadarmaki, Hossein Mahmoudian, Gholamreza Jamshidiha, and Mohammad Abdelahad. Assistance and support from Evelien Bakker and Bernadette Deelen at Springer are greatly appreciated. Their patience and support contributed greatly to the quality of the book as with the extension of their deadline we were able to add more chapters and new findings into the book. Finally, we would like to appreciate our families for their continuing support over the last several years enabling us to complete this book.

Contents

List of Tables

List of Figures

About the Authors

Mohammad Jalal Abbasi-Shavazi is Associate Professor of the Department of Demography, University of Tehran (UT); and Adjunct Fellow, Australian Demographic and Social Research Institute (ADSRI), The Australian National University (ANU). He completed his Ph.D. and a 2 year Postdoctoral Fellowship at the ANU Demography Program during 1994–2000. He was the Head of the Department of Demography of the UT during 2002–2006, and has been the Chair of the Division of Population Research of the UT since 2001. He has been elected Vice-President of the Asian Population Association (APA). His main research has been focused on fertility, and he has completed several studies on Iranian fertility transition, the results of which have been presented at national and international population conferences, and published in leading demographic journals. Abbasi-Shavazi's contribution to the understanding of the fall of fertility in Iran during the last three decades is widely acknowledged. In addition to fertility, he has published papers on family patterns and transformation as well as consanguinity in Iran in various journals, and has also worked on other areas including reproductive health/infertility, immigration in Australia, and Afghan refugees in Iran.

Peter McDonald is Professor of Demography and Director of the Australian Demographic and Social Research Institute at the Australian National University. He has been elected Vice President (2006–2009) and President (2010–2013) of the International Union for the Scientific Study of Population, the international association of professional demographers. McDonald was Head of Research at the Australian Institute of Family Studies for a period of 11 years during the 1980s and 1990s. He has written extensively on the demography of the family in both developed and developing country settings and on theory related to family change. Besides Australia, he is frequently consulted on the issue of population futures (causes, consequences and policies) by governments around the world, especially in Europe and East Asia. He is a leading expert on policies, including labour supply policies, for countries facing very low fertility rates. He has been highly influential in work and family policy and labour supply futures policy. His theoretical work on the causes of very low fertility rates is widely cited in academic papers and meetings and acknowledged by governments around the world that are addressing the problems associated with very low fertility rates.

Meimanat Hosseini-Chavoshi is a Senior Officer of the Family Health and Population Department of the Iran Ministry of Health and Medical Education, & Research Associate at ADSRI, ANU. She completed her MA and Ph.D. in Demography at the ANU. Hosseini's Ph.D. thesis was focused on fertility regulation in Iran. Hosseini-Chavoshi has worked with the Iran Ministry of Health for more than two decades. She has worked in the area of family planning and reproductive health at both provincial and national levels, and has been the focal person in the design, implementation and data analysis of several national KAP surveys during the 1990s as well as the 2000 Iran Demographic and Health Survey. She is expert in survey design and data analysis, and has a long experience on reproductive health and population programs in Iran. She is now a member of the Scientific Committee of the currently planned 2009 IDHS. Hosseini-Chavoshi has been collaborating with Abbasi and McDonald in studies of fertility transition in Iran since 2002.

Chapter 1
The Fall in Iranian Fertility: Theoretical Considerations

Confounding all conventional wisdom, the fertility rate in the Islamic Republic of Iran fell from 7.0 births per woman in 1979 to 1.9 births per woman in 2006. That this, the largest and fastest fall in fertility ever recorded, should have occurred in one of the worlds few Islamic Republics demands explanation. This is the purpose of this book.

Conventional wisdom has been that falls in fertility in developing countries are gained slowly and only in open societies, particularly those open to the western notion that rapid population growth is an obstacle to economic development. The western package of development, promoted by organizations such as the World Bank and the International Monetary Fund, combines economic reforms including abolition of tariffs, removal of currency controls, private foreign investment, transfer of technology and human capital enhancement with aggressive, government-sponsored family planning programs. Japan provided the first apparent evidence of the appropriateness of this development model and it was followed by other Asian success stories such as South Korea, Singapore, Thailand and Indonesia (Jones and Leete 2002; Jones and Karim 2005; Robinson and Ross 2007). The Islamic Revolution ensured that this western package was not implemented in Iran yet fertility has fallen just as fast if not faster than in those countries where the package was applied. In this book, we address how this occurred.

Before and After the Islamic Revolution

Under western influence, Mohammad Reza Shah's Iran moved down the western path of deve-lopment in the 1960s but progress was slow. In an Iran made wealthy by the oil-boom, the fertility rate hovered around six children per woman throughout the 1970s and the economy remained centralised and stagnant. In contrast, the oil boom signalled the beginning of a consistent fall in fertility in Indonesia and major economic reforms. The 1970s oil boom in Iran put vast financial resources in the hands of the State but this served only to entrench the pre-existing state capitalism. Investment was

M.J. Abbasi-Shavazi et al., *The Fertility Transition in Iran: Revolution and Reproduction*,

channelled into state-organised forms of import substitution especially in agriculture and manufacturing. At the end of the Shah's regime, the state sector comprised 43% of Gross National Product (Richards and Waterbury 1998).

By the end of the 1970s, most Iranians considered that their country was wealthy but that they themselves were not seeing the fruits of that wealth. The outcome was regime change through popular revolution, the only example of such change in the Middle East in the past 40 years. The strong and viable alternative at the time was an Islamic Republic. Iran became a state with a new constitution in which all legislation passed by parliament must be reviewed by a Guardianship Council before being enacted. The Council of leading Muslim clerics evaluates legislation against sharia law and the Republic's constitution. Reform in the new republic was focussed first and foremost on the application of a conservative social and religious regime and upon the realignment of foreign relationships.

Highly visible were reforms related to women including the application of their status as contingent upon a responsible male, separation of the sexes in public, the enforcement of the strict dress code and the lowering of the minimum age at marriage for girls and boys from 15 and 18 to 13 and 15 years, respectively (Azimi 1981).[1] The family planning program that had enjoyed only modest success at best was allowed to fall into disrepair and contraception became less readily available. Indeed, the new regime, plunged almost immediately into a long and bloody war with Iraq, adopted a number of pronatalist measures (Chapter 2). Rejection of western values and isolation from those values along with the changes in women's status portrayed Iran to the West as being culturally conservative, especially in relation to fertility and family planning. This was borne out in the first years of the regime through increases in fertility rates across the country. In some provinces, especially those with substantial ethnic minorities, fertility rose in the first half of the 1980s to almost nine children per woman.

In contrast to the radical nature of social reform, economic reform was very limited in the new republic. Stimulated by the war and perhaps by the Islamic approach to economic development, industry became even more state-centralised and isolated from world markets. Richards and Waterbury (1998, p. 241–3) reported that, in the aftermath of the revolution, 580 large to medium sized companies were nationalized. Protection, inflation and currency mismanagement were rampant. Employment creation (mainly in the public sector) did not keep up with growth in the labour supply, income per capita in 1992 was 38 percent lower than it had been in 1979 and more than two-thirds of new jobs created in the same period were in the public sector. In the early 1990s, public enterprises accounted for 72% of all employment and the free market price of foreign exchange was twenty times higher than the official rate. The demands of the war, while benefiting a minority involved in the support of the war effort, left the economic circumstances of the majority in decline and led to the entire depletion of accumulated reserves. The hopes of most

[1] Marriage for girls aged 9 to 12 was possible subject to their physical ability, medical approval, and legal permission from the court.

people that their economic circumstances would be greatly improved through regime change were not realised.

On the other hand, the new government invested heavily in infrastructure especially electricity and water supply. More importantly for the story of this book was the creation throughout the country of widespread and cheap access to education and health services. Infant and child mortality rates fell sharply and education and literacy rose rapidly. Furthermore, despite the restrictions placed upon women in many areas of their lives, the egalitarian nature of the revolution extended full access to education and health services to women. Iranian girls and women spent more years in school and university than was the case previously (Abdollahyan 2004; Shadi-Talab 2005). Adult literacy classes were provided for those who were illiterate, including women. As a result, the levels of education of women of reproductive ages have increased substantially over the last four decades, and the education gap between rural and urban areas has narrowed considerably (Abbasi-Shavazi 2002 p. 437). In this respect, the revolution was highly enlightened compared, for example, to what was to happen under the Taliban regime in neighbouring Afghanistan.

The election of the Khatami government in 1997 and its re-election in 2001 signalled a new era of democratisation and liberalisation. This era consolidated social changes that had already taken place and created an expectation of further change. Overall, however, despite strong popular support, further liberalisation was slow during the Khatami years. Nevertheless, through the rapid expansion of education, especially women's education, the revolution has given rise to forces that in time may modify the course of the revolution itself. Low fertility itself frees women to consider non-familial roles, roles that are much more likely to be pursued through the enlightenment brought by education (McDonald 2000a, b).

There has been a series of meetings at the Ministry of Health since 2000 to discuss revision of population policy in Iran. Regional population policies have been considered as many provinces are experiencing below replacement fertility. It has also been suggested to establish or revive the national population council. However, as yet, the issue has not been taken up by the high-ranking officials.

In October 2006, at a joint meeting with government officials and Members of Parliament, Iran's president, Mahmoud Ahmadinejad, defended an increasing population growth rate and called for a baby boom to almost double the country's population to 120 million. He told MPs that women should work less and devote more time to their main mission of raising children. Ahmadinejad said: 'I am against saying that two children are enough. Our country has a lot of capacity. It has the capacity for many children to grow in it. It even has the capacity for 120 million people. Westerners have got problems. Because their population growth is negative, they are worried and fear that if our population increases, we will triumph over them'.

Ahmadinejad's statement was criticized by many scholars and newspapers. There was also resistance from within the government and the Ministry of Health and Medical Education, in particular. In response to these criticisms, a Government spokesman said that the President did not mean to change the policy but his view is that population growth is not worrying and our country has the capacity to respond to the needs of the people. In brief, Ahmadinejads statement while based on the current population situation in Iran, is considered to be mainly a political statement as he referred to reproductive health policy as a western agenda.

The Watershed in 1986

The year, 1986, constituted something of a watershed in the demographic history of Iran. In that year, the oil price plummeted greatly reducing the revenues of the government, the war was in its 6 year with no sign of resolution and the Islamic Republics first census revealed the massive growth of population and the high fertility rates that had applied in the first years of the revolution. The populace had had 6 years to realise that their economic aspirations were not about to be met and, with the fall in the oil price, a worsening of their circumstances was much more likely. Our analysis (Chapter 3) shows that the fertility rate began its sustained fall around this time.

The 1986 Census revealed that the 1976–86 intercensal growth rate of population had been almost 4% per annum and that a huge cohort of children had been created. For a country that had always struggled in finding work for its burgeoning numbers of young people, the future challenge was immense especially in the light of the fiscal turnaround caused by the fall in the oil price. A series of meetings was held in the following few years that led eventually to the reinstatement of the national family planning program and its support by Iran's religious leaders including the supreme leader, Ayatollah Khomeini (see Chapter 2 for more details).

Acceptance of the Reality of Fertility Decline

Some smaller-scale surveys were undertaken in the early 1990s that indicated surprisingly high use of contraception and that fertility was falling (Malekafzali 1992; Abbasi-Shavazi et al. 2002). However, there was widespread scepticism about the accuracy of the results of these surveys within Iran and, even more so, outside of Iran. Iran was seen as a country in which there was a culture of high fertility, a conservative Muslim government, subjugation of women, a poorly performing economy and isolation from the West. By conventional wisdom, fertility does not fall in such circumstances.

Substantial fertility decline in Iran was not factored into the projections of the United Nations Population Division until the 1998 round of projections,[2] and was not fully accepted until the presentation of Abbasi-Shavazi's estimates based on the 1996 Census at conferences of the International Union for the Scientific Study of Population held in Bangladesh in January 2000 (Abbasi-Shavazi 2000) and in

[2] Ladier-Fouladi's (1997) paper was influential in this regard.

Tokyo in March 2001 (Abbasi-Shavazi 2001). The 1976–96 fertility trends revealed by the 1996 Census have been confirmed by the large scale 2000 Demographic and Health Survey (IDHS), the 2002 Iran Fertility Transition Survey (IFTS), and the 2006 Census. These data also indicated continued falls in fertility to levels below replacement in several provinces (Chapter 3) and very high levels of contraceptive prevalence. There can no longer be any doubt that a remarkable transformation in Iranian fertility has occurred. This book seeks to provide an understanding of how this happened against the expectations of most demographers.

Theoretical Considerations

The physical reproduction of the group is fundamental to all societies. It is not surprising therefore that changes in fertility rates have been associated with a wide range of socio-cultural and economic factors. The main theoretical positions are outlined here with some cursory consideration given to their applicability in the Iranian fertility transition. In subsequent chapters, the applicability of these theories is considered in more detail.

Any proposed theoretical explanation of fertility decline must be operationalised through the so-called proximate determinants of fertility. These are essentially conditions that effect whether or not a woman will have a live birth. Based on an original formulation by Davis and Blake (1956), Bongaarts (1978) and Bongaarts and Potter (1983) specified the proximate determinants to include being in a sexual union, being sexually active, breastfeeding and lactational amenorrhea, use of contraception, abortion, foetal loss, natural infertility and pathological infertility. Of these, in theory, only three could have been involved in the massive fall of fertility that has been observed in Iran: being in a sexual union (age at marriage and the proportion ever marrying), contraception and abortion. The relevance of each of these three factors is considered in the subsequent chapters.

Demographic Transition Theory: Modernisation, Industrialisation, Urbanisation

Thompson (1929), writing near the end of the European fertility transition, attributed the decline in fertility that had occurred in the previous 60 years to the social and economic forces of modern society. This description became known as demographic transition theory under the authorship of Frank Notestein (1945, 1953). Notestein's 1953 paper attributed the transition to several broad social and economic changes including a loosening of the hold of traditional forces, the advance of education and rational thought, changes in the economic benefits and costs of children and the emergence of new economic roles for women that were incompatible with childbearing. Many other formulations of transition theory have followed. These have been well reviewed in other places (e.g., McDonald 1993; Hirschman 1994; Mason 1997; Szreter 1993; Kirk 1996), but it is worth noting Hirschmans observation that transition theory has room for every causal variable (Hirschman 1994, p. 211).

Most of the conditions of change included in classic demographic transition theory do not apply to the Iranian transition and it is for this reason that demographers were highly sceptical that the fall in fertility in Iran was real. The Islamic Revolution represented a reassertion of the hold of traditional forces and led to a reversal of new emerging economic roles for women. In the West, the Iranian revolution was perceived as the antithesis of modernization. Advances in industrialization have been small during the transition years, 1986–2000. On the other hand, urbanization has proceeded apace and education levels have risen substantially.

Improvements in Child Survival

Demographic transition theory also included the important proviso that fertility would not fall unless preceded or accompanied by a fall in child mortality. It has been argued that, prior to the transition, high infant and child mortality rates promoted high fertility rates because the interests of households were in the number of children who survived rather than in the number who were born. Higher rates of child survival figured prominently in Davis's (1963) formulation of demographic transition as multi-phasic response. Its importance was reasserted in a paper by Cleland (2001a). He suggests that the main pathway through which improvements in child survival contribute to fertility decline is explicitly economic: the pressure on families of having to rear abnormally large numbers of surviving children (Cleland 2001a, p. 87). Others argue that where the concern is to produce a given number of surviving children or surviving sons to ensure the future wellbeing of the parents, this can be done with fewer births if parents have confidence that their children will survive to adulthood (Wilson and Airey 1999).

In regard to Iran, the very high fertility rates of the early 1980s would indeed have led to abnormally large numbers of surviving children especially given the falls in child mortality that resulted from the provision of basic health services for all during the years of the revolutionary government (see Chapter 2).

Demand Theory

Within the more rigorous framework of economics, demand theory argues straightforwardly that fertility falls when the costs of an additional child exceed the benefits of having that child (Easterlin 1975; Easterlin and Crimmins 1985; Leibenstein 1974, 1975; Becker 1991; Becker et al. 1990). The principal focus of demand theory is that, under new conditions, the costs of children increase and, in the process, for many people, surpass the economic and psychic values attached to having an additional child. The new conditions that may give rise to increased costs of children are numerous. As employment becomes based upon a modern, industrial economy as distinct from agrarian family production, parents must invest more on each child in order that the child will be able to compete in the new labour market. Where there are large cohorts of young people, as in societies with past high levels of fertility, the perceived need to invest in the quality of children compared to their quantity takes on a greater imperative. While, in more gender-segregated societies, this need for investment may be perceived as being more important for boy children, parents also need to invest in quality girl children so that they are more able to compete in the marriage market. The modern, industrialised economy also produces more expensive and diversified must-have goods for children, so that children become more expensive. Children may also become more expensive relative to other goods and services and, where it is considered that a couple already have sufficient children, access to these goods and services may be more appealing than the marginal additional child. In societies where the employment of women in the paid labour market is advanced, additional time spent in childbearing and child rearing reduces the woman's capacity to earn income. The demand theory of fertility decline has been criticized by scholars (Cleland and Wilson 1987; Robinson 1997) essentially on the grounds that parents are unlikely to make precise econometric calculations in making their decisions about children. However, it is still possible to postulate that a generalised sense or understanding that too many children will lower the economic standard of the family may affect decisions about having children.

Within the demand theory framework, Caldwell (1982, 2006) has argued that, the rise of mass education produced a reversal of the direction of the flow of wealth between parents and children. As a result, instead of being an economic asset to parents through their labour, children became an economic liability. Caldwell postulated three demand-related mechanisms through which mass education changes the flow of wealth between parents and children: reduction of the child's potential as a worker, increased schooling costs, and the fact that schooling makes the child more dependent. However, beyond demand theory, he also suggested that education is the gateway to cultural change and to the introduction of Western values that impact on fertility.

It is not possible in this study of Iran, and maybe it is never possible, to make exact calculations of the costs and benefits of having children for a family. However, it is possible to argue that the very large family sizes that followed the revolution, certainly questioned in the mid-1980s at the national level for economic reasons, were also questioned by individual families for economic reasons.

Economic Expectations and Economic Realities

Demand theory is based on a cross-sectional comparison of the costs and benefits of having an additional child (the decision at the margin). However, decision making about children relates to the long-term, economic futures of families. Central to such decision-making will be the economic aspirations of couples. If an association is drawn between numbers of children and the capacity to realise economic expectations, the number of children may be controlled to a greater extent than a cross-sectional demand theory analysis would predict (Casterline 2001a). It is highly conventional for Western-influenced family planning programs to draw this association in their publicity. Emphasis is placed upon the small, prosperous and healthy family. We have argued above that the oil wealth generated in the 1970s engendered high economic expectations among Iranians, but that a large gulf between expectations and reality has continued to the present day. In this book, using data from the Iran Fertility Transition Survey, we investigate the extent to which Iranians have drawn an association between numbers of children and the realisation of their economic aspirations (Chapter 8).

It is arguable also that the level of motivation generated by economic aspirations will be greater in societies in which people have the perception that economic and social mobility are possible. Where societal structures inhibit social and economic mobility, there is much less reason to strive for economic improvement. The Islamic revolution was at least partly founded on the pursuit of economic equity and egalitarianism and, following the success of the revolution, the people of Iran were open to the proliferation of merit-based social mobility.

Status Enhancement

Related to the desire to improve economic wellbeing is the desire to enhance one's social standing in the community. Kasarda and Billy (1985), Kasarda et al. (1986) have postulated that couples may restrict the number of their children because fewer children will mean that they will have the energy and capital that will enable them to rise up the social ladder of success. This argument may also extend to the desire to improve the social standing of one's children by parents being able to invest more in each child if their number is few. In a religious, egalitarian society such as Iran, the main means to rise to a position of social importance are through religious organisations and through education. The chance of increasing ones status through entrepreneurial activity is present but not prominent. For most Iranians, their education level is already in place before they have their children and, to a large extent, this is also true of other pathways to social importance. Thus, the opportunity to enhance one's own social standing through having fewer children is likely to be relatively limited in Iran. On the other hand, Iranian parents have very strong motivations to enhance their children's position in society.

Culture, Religion and the State: the Institutional Perspective

There are those who argue that changes in economic structures or changes in knowledge and ideas occur mainly through changes in social, economic, religious and political institutions (McNicoll 1980, 1985, 1994). Social institutions may be interpreted as the socially constructed (and sanctioned) rules that provide solutions to recurrent problems of individual action and interaction (McNicoll 1985). In this theme, Greenhalgh (1988, p. 630) states:

> to understand the causes and character of fertility decline, we need a society-specific institutional approach. [An approach] that focuses on the political, economic, and social institutions [...] within which demographic decision making and behaviour occur.

Culture or institutions are seen conventionally as conservative forces, that is, forces that serve to maintain the status quo. Cultural institutions define the identity of a people and as such will only change slowly, or, as occurred in Iran in 1979, in a revolutionary way. Furthermore, culture connected to the family (reproduction) is likely to be even slower to change than, say, culture related to farming practice or to business arrangements (McDonald 1994; Abbasi-Shavazi and McDonald 2007). It is almost certainly the case that initial incredulity relating to the fall in fertility in Iran was driven by the sense that cultural supports to high fertility were strong and resilient in Iran, especially after the revolution. Essentially, there was disbelief that a conservative Muslim society that had isolated itself from the West could experience a sharp fall in fertility. The fact that this fall did occur means that an explanation is required of how the conservative cultural institutions of Iran, especially the religious institutions, were tolerant or accepting of this change. Most important in this regard was the creation of a national family planning program that was accessible to all. This is addressed in Chapter 2. Access to the means to control fertility is an obviously necessary component of any fertility decline. Also, in a country in which sexual relationships outside marriage are subject to very severe sanctions, the institution of marriage (through age at marriage and the proportion marrying) can also be an important determinant of the fertility trend. This is considered in Chapter 5.

Finally, institutional change in relation to education must always be considered in explaining any fertility transition. This is especially the case in Iran where, following the revolution, access to education was extended widely across the country, especially in rural areas. Education provides access to the modern world and its ideas and it provides its holders with the capability and confidence to make their own decisions. Education figures prominently in most explanations of fertility decline.

Gender Equity Theory

McDonald (2000a, b) has argued that fertility does not decline without a change in the standing of women within the household. He argues that all fertility declines are associated with a change in the nature of the husband–wife relationship that affords greater standing to the wife than is the case in most patriarchal traditional societies. Reduction of fertility involves cooperation between husbands and wives, often at the instigation of the wife. Women can gain this greater equity within the marital relationship through contact with other women and with social institutions beyond the family circle such as modern health systems, family planning programs and the schools of their children. In time, advancing education of both women and their husbands becomes the essential driving force. It provides women with access to modern institutions and ideas and with the confidence to relate to their husbands as a partner rather than as a vassal. Together, the status of the young couple is enhanced relative to that of the older generation because it is the young, educated couple that has access to the new technology and new ideas that define the future. Finally, urbanisation and its often-consequent nuclearisation of the family promotes the independence of the young couple and hence a higher degree of gender equity within the relationship. McDonald argues that women's status within the household can change considerably although there may be little change in their roles outside the family, especially in relation to labour force participation.

Implicit in gender equity theory is the idea that, prior to fertility decline, many women are having more children than they want, that there is an unmet demand for contraception. This is supported by the fact that, in all fertility declines, it is the very large family sizes that start to disappear first. There is certainly a question as to why women would want to subject themselves to the burden and risk of numerous pregnancies long after they had fulfilled even the most demanding family size requirements.

Iran exemplifies the pre-conditions of this theory. Education levels of women have risen dramatically in a very short time frame throughout the country, including the literacy levels of women beyond school age. In addition, women have been able to engage relatively freely with other women and with institutions such as the health system and the education system. At the same time, their involvement in paid employment has remained very restricted (Chapter 9).

Diffusion of New Values, Rational Thought, Westernisation, Ideation

Modernization and economic change as determinants of fertility transition have been rejected by some scholars (Lesthaeghe and Wilson 1986; Cleland and Wilson 1987). Based on the findings of the European Fertility Project and observation of the transitions in many developing countries, they have argued that fertility decline is produced by diffusion of new ideas and knowledge about fertility regulation rather than by changes in socio-economic factors or social institutions. Like the fork and the potato, contraception is a good idea that has found its time (Cleland 2001b). In the case of Europe in the nineteenth century, the theory that increased use of fertility control was due to gradual diffusion of new ideas was linked to the view that there was a contemporaneous rise in rational or secular thought (as opposed to religion) through the transfer of ideas from more secular societies to more traditional societies. In modern times, the role of the mass media and government-sponsored family planning programmes in the diffusion of the idea of contraception (Hornik and McAnany 2001) has been emphasised. It is also argued that westernisation (the adoption of western values or ideas) has been a part of this process (Caldwell 1982). Diffusion or ideational theory has spawned complex models of the processes of the spread of ideas through social learning, influences and networks (Montgomery and Casterline 1996).

The key question in this theoretical framework is whether diffusion of new ideas is sufficient in itself as an explanation of fertility decline or whether diffusion must be associated with other societal changes (Casterline 2001b). Are new users of contraception passive receptors of new ideas or are they active participants motivated by the circumstances in which they live and their aspirations for the future? As contraception operates to reduce fertility at the level of the individual couple, it is pure logic that diffusion of the idea of contraception must be part of the process. It is also logical that efficient means to diffuse and deliver contraception, such as government-sponsored family planning programs, will speed the process. Propaganda and overt or subtle coercion associated with family planning programmes are also very likely to be successful diffusion mechanisms so long as there is no social reaction. Once the idea of smaller family size is firmly established, relaxation of coercive approaches is very unlikely to lead to a return to high fertility.

A relatively unsuccessful family planning program was in operation in Iran prior to the Islamic revolution. Compared to Indonesia (Hull and Mosely 2009; Hull and Hull, 1984; Hugo et al. 1987), for example, Iran at the end of the 1970s had higher levels of education and a higher level of economic development and urbanisation, yet, its family planning program was much less effective (Moore 2007). Following the revolution, the pronatalist approach of the new regime was adopted enthusiastically, perhaps motivated in part by the impacts of the Iran–Iraq war and the more generalised sense of threat from beyond its borders. Yet, by 1986, well before the recommencement of the family planning program in 1989, fertility began to fall steadily (Chapter 3). In 1986, the West remained despised and copying of its ways could not have been an explanation of the fertility decline, although it may be argued that the later adoption of a national family planning program was modelled on experience in other countries such as Indonesia. There is also little evidence that the family planning program, once adopted, was coercive or even that it was characterised by major propaganda campaigns. Targets and local-level shaming techniques, successful in Indonesia (Hull 2007), also seem to have played little part in the widespread adoption of family planning in Iran. Thus, the diffusion theory of fertility decline seems to have much less substance at the macro-level in the Iranian case than in most other countries. The story seems to be more of diffusion at the micro-level. The revolutionary government had previously created an efficient, accessible public health system (Chapter 2). Once an efficient family planning program was attached to this pre-existing system, it was adopted through local diffusion mechanisms led by the female, base-level health worker (*behvarz*). That this local level approach could be successful in every corner of the country suggests that there were stronger motivating forces than simply the personality of the *behvarz*.

The Tempo and Quantum of Childbearing

The measure of annual fertility conventionally used in studies such as this one, the total fertility rate, is subject to fluctuations from year to year because of changes in the timing of births (tempo) rather than changes in the number of births that women eventually have during their lifetime (quantum). It is quite likely that the very high fertility in the early years following the revolution was affected by a shortening of birth intervals (births being brought forward in time). This possibility is investigated in Chapter 4 through the use of parity progression analysis. A tempo-induced increase in fertility can be expected to be followed by a fall because people have already had most of the children that they want to have. The decline in fertility in Iran from 1986 may have been due at least partly to this process.

Fertility declines in several countries have been interpreted as being driven initially by changes in age at first marriage that, in turn, lead to changes in the tempo of fertility through delay of the first birth. While it has been suggested that fertility might rise in the future when the rise in age at first marriage ceases, there have been few if any instances of this actually occurring. However, again, parity progression analysis and study of the marriage trends will be used to investigate this possibility in Iran. In general, rises in age at first marriage in Iran have been small (Chapter 5) given the very large increases in education for both men and women. Thus, while there may be some element of a tempo effect deriving from delay of the first birth, its effect on overall fertility decline is likely to be modest. We show in Chapter 4, however, that Iranian couples have developed a very long interval between the first and the second birth and this would also have a tempo effect on the period total fertility rate.

Discussion

The analysis of historical fertility declines has spawned numerous theoretical explanations as described above. While fertility decline is becoming ubiquitous occurring in country after country, this does not mean that a totally common explanation needs to be found that is applicable in all cases. The central argument against this notion is that fertility decline has occurred in societies that differ dramatically at the onset of the decline in terms of economic development, political and social structure, family organization, education levels, women's status, child survival, social diffusion mechanisms, contraceptive technology and availability and the level of government commitment to fertility reduction. Inevitably, therefore, the story will vary from place to place and across different periods of time. Nevertheless, there will be common themes and it is to these that we turn our attention in the following chapters of the book. There is no question that the case of fertility reduction in Iran is unusual and as such it presents challenges to conventional theories.

Appendix 1.1: Data Sources

The data sources employed in the study provide measures of the impact of the more important proximate determinants of fertility including nuptiality and contraception (Lucas 1994). The data used in this study are drawn from the 1986, 1996 and 2006 Censuses, the 2000 Iran Demographic and Health Survey (IDHS), the 2002 Iran

Fertility Transition Survey (IFTS) and the 2005 Iran Low Fertility Survey. Descriptions of the three survey sources follow. Census data are used mainly in Chapters 3 and 5.

The 2000 Iran Demographic and Health Survey

The IDHS was conducted in October 2000 by the Ministry of Health. Using the 1996 Census framework and the systematic cluster stratification sampling method, members of 111,989 households were successfully interviewed. The sample size of IDHS was optimised to enable most fertility and reproductive health indices to be estimated at the provincial level. It was designed so that in each of 27 provinces, 4,000 households (2,000 households equally in each rural and urban area) were interviewed with the exception that in Tehran province, 2,000 households exclusively in Tehran City were interviewed. The response rate was very high (97.9%). A total of 90,924 women were successfully interviewed about their reproductive life and behaviour. The data set is very rich in demonstrating cross-sectional fertility and contraceptive use by different demographic and social characteristics at the time of the survey in 2000, as well as the parity progression ratios during the reproductive life of women. However, it does not allow the matching of contraceptive use and fertility behaviour during a woman's reproductive life, that is, how a woman regulates her reproductive fertility during her reproductive years. This is the main source of data for Chapters 4 and 6.

The 2002 Iran Fertility Transition Survey

The 2002 Iran Fertility Transition Survey (IFTS) was a Wellcome Trust funded project conducted by MJ Abbasi-Shavazi and P. McDonald with the third author's collaboration in April 2002 in four selected provinces of Iran namely Gilan, West Azarbaijan, Yazd and Sistan and Baluchistan. This study used the IDHS sampling frame and re-interviewed half of the women who had been interviewed in IDHS. The aim of this survey was to assess recent trends and differences in fertility in order to understand the phenomenon of fertility decline in Iran. A total of 5,190 ever-married-women aged 15–49 women were re-interviewed. This survey reveals strong contrasts in terms of socio-cultural, religious as well as demographic patterns between each province, and is representative of the heterogeneity of Iran. This is the only data set that allows various aspects of fertility to be examined according to cultural factors such as religion and ethnicity. These data are utilised mainly in Chapters 8 and 9.

The 2005 Iran Low Fertility Survey

The Iran Low Fertility Survey (ILFS) was also conducted by M.J. Abbasi-Shavazi and P. McDonald with the third author's collaboration during April–May 2005 through an award from the Wellcome Trust. The general aim of the ILFS was to investigate the health and social consequences of early cessation of childbearing in Iran. The survey was specifically designed to enable detailed in-depth analysis of contraceptive use and fertility behaviour and to show how women have regulated their fertility during their reproductive lives using contraception to delay or limit their fertility. A comprehensive life history questionnaire was used to obtain information simultaneously about the respondents' pregnancy history and contraceptive use history.

The survey was conducted in the three provinces of Yazd, Isfahan, Gilan, and the greater city of Tehran. A sample of 7,350 households was approached, and 5,526 ever-married women aged 15–54 were interviewed. This survey is the main source of data for Chapter 7 and is used extensively in Chapters 4 and 6. These provinces were selected because of their low fertility levels compared with other provinces and because the age at last birth is very low in these provinces in comparison with other provinces in Iran. More than half of women in these provinces cease childbearing by their late 20s (Hosseini-Chavoshi et al. 2006).

The two provinces of Tehran and Isfahan are among the most populous provinces of Iran, and their contribution to Iranian population growth is substantial. Tehran is the capital of Iran with a population of around 12 million and is a multicultural society hosting a large number of migrants from all over Iran. Isfahan, located in the centre of Iran, is populated by Persians, and is one of the main tourist attractions in Iran and a trading centre. These provinces also enjoy high socio-economic characteristics and are regarded as the developed provinces in Iran, thus their fertility trends and patterns may be replicated in other provinces as they become more developed. Also, each selected province is identified with a particular culture in Iran. Gilan province, located in the North, has a developed farming economy and has recorded the lowest fertility among all provinces in Iran. People in Gilan speak Gilaki (a dialect), and are characterised as having a liberal view toward life (Abbasi-Shavazi et al. 2004). Yazd also enjoys high levels of socio-economic development and is located in the centre of Iran. Both Isfahan and Yazd have a conservative religious culture, despite their high levels of development.

References

Abbasi-Shavazi, MJ (2000) National trends and social inclusion: fertility trends and differentials in the Islamic republic of Iran, 1972–1996, paper presented at the IUSSP conference on family planning in the 21st century, Dhaka, 16–21 January

Abbasi-Shavazi MJ (2001) Below replacement fertility in Iran: progress and prospects, paper presented at the workshop on low fertility in advanced countries: trends, theories and policies, Tokyo, 21–23 March, 2001

Abbasi-Shavazi MJ (2002) Recent changes and the future of fertility in Iran. In: United Nations Population Division, completing the fertility transition, New York, pp 425–439

Abbasi-Shavazi MJ, McDonald P (2007) Family change in Iran: religion, revolution, and the state. In: Jayakody A, Thornton A, Axinn W (eds) International family change: ideational perspectives. Lawrence Erlbaum Associates, New York, pp 177–198

Abbasi-Shavazi MJ, Mehryar AH, Jones G, McDonald P (2002) Revolution, war and modernisation: population policy and fertility change in Iran. J Popul Res 19(1):25–46

Abbasi-Shavazi MJ, Hosseini-Chavoshi M, McDonald PF, Delavar B (2004) Fertility transition in Iran: evidence from four selected provinces (Persian). Ministry of Health and Medical Education, Tehran

Abdollahyan H (2004) The generations gap in contemporary Iran. J Welt Trends 44:78–85

Azimi H (1981) Population growth and its needs. Budget and Planning Organization (Persian), Department of Human Resources and Social Planning, Tehran

Becker G (1991) A treatise on the family, Enlargedth edn. Harvard University Press, Cambridge

Becker G, Murphy KM, Tamura RF (1990) Human capital, fertility and economic growth. J Political Econ 98:12–37

Bongaarts J (1978) A framework for analysing the proximate determinants of fertility. Popul Dev Rev 1(2):298–296

Bongaarts J, Potter RG (1983) Fertility, biology, and behavior: an analysis of the proximate determinants. Academic, New York

Caldwell J (1982) Theory of fertility decline. Academic, London

Caldwell J (2006) Demographic transition theory. Springer, Dordrecht

Casterline J (2001a) The pace of fertility transition: national patterns in the second half of the twentieth century. In: Bulatao R, Casterline J (eds) Global fertility transition. A supplement to Pop Dev Rev 27. Population Council, New York, pp 17–52

Casterline J (2001b) Diffusion processes and fertility transition: introduction. In: Casterline J (ed) Diffusion processes and fertility transition, selected perspectives, Committee on Population, National Research Council. National Academy Press, Washington, D.C., pp 1–38

Cleland J (2001a) The effects of improved survival on fertility: a reassessment. In: Bulatao R, Casterline J (eds) Global fertility transition. A supplement to Popul Dev Rev 27. Population Council, New York, pp 60–92

Cleland J (2001b) Potatoes and pills: an overview of innovation-diffusion contributions to explanations of fertility decline. In: Casterline J (ed) Diffusion processes and fertility transition, selected perspectives, Committee on Population, National Research Council. National Academy Press, Washington, D.C., pp 39–65

Cleland J, Wilson C (1987) Demand theories of the fertility transition: an iconoclastic view. Popul Stud 41(1):5–30

Davis K (1963) The theory of change and response in modern demographic history. Popul Index 29(4):345–366

Davis K, Blake J (1956) Social structure and fertility. Econ Dev Cultur Change 4:211–235

Easterlin R (1975) An economic framework for fertility analysis. Stud Fam Plann 6(1):54–63

Easterlin R, Crimmins E (1985) The fertility revolution. University of Chicago Press, Chicago, IL

Greenhalgh S (1988) Fertility as mobility: sinic transitions. Popul Dev Rev 14(4):629–674

Hirschman C (1994) Why fertility changes. Annu Rev Sociol 20:203–233

Hugo G, Hull TH, Hull V, Jones G (1987) Demographic dimensions of Indonesian development. Oxford in Asia, Kuala Lumpur

Hull TH (2007). Formative years of family planning in Indonesia. In: Robinson WA, Ross JA (eds) The global family planning revolution. The World Bank (electronic), Washington, D.C., Chapter 15, pp 235–256

Hull TH, Hull VJ (1984) Population change in Indonesia: findings of the 1980 census. Bull Indones Econ Stud 20(3):95–119

Hull TH, Mosely H (2009) Revitalization of family planning in Indonesia. The Government of Indonesia and the United Nations Population Funds, Jakarta

Hornik R and McAnany C (2001) Mass media and fertility change. In: Casterline J (ed) Diffusion processes and fertility transition, selected perspectives, Committee on Population, National Research Council. National Academy Press, Washington, D.C., pp 208–239

Hosseini-Chavoshi M, McDonald P, Abbasi-Shavazi MJ (2006) The Iranian Fertility Decline, 1981–1999: An application of the synthetic parity progression ratio method. Population 61(5–6):701–718

Jones GW, Leete R (2002) Asia's family planning programs as low fertility is attained. Stud Fam Plann 33(1):114–126
Jones G, Karim M (2005) Islam, the state and population, Hurst and Co., London
Kasarda JD, Billy JOC (1985) Social mobility and fertility. Annu Rev Sociol 11:305–328
Kasarda JD, Billy JOC, West K (1986) Status enhancement and fertility: reproductive responses to social mobility and educational opportunity. Academic, Orlando, FL
Kirk D (1996) Demographic transition theory. Popul Stud 50(3):361–387
Ladier-Fouladi M (1997) The fertility transition in Iran. Popul: Engl Sel 9:191–214
Leibenstein H (1974) An interpretation of the economic theory of fertility: promising path or blind alley? J Econ Lit 12(2):457–479
Leibenstein H (1975) The economic theory of fertility decline. Q J Econ 89(1):1–39
Lesthaeghe R, Wilson C (1986) Modes of production, secularization, and the pace of fertility decline in Western Europe, 1870–1930. In: Coale A, Watkins S (eds) The decline of fertility in Europe. Princeton University Press, Princeton, NJ, pp 261–292
Lucas D (1994) The proximate determinants of fertility. In: Lucas D, Meyer P (eds) Beginning population studies. The Australian National University, Canberra
Malekafzali H (1992) Population and Family Planning Programs in the Islamic Republic of Iran [Persian], Nabz J Contin Educ 2:3–7
Mason K (1997) Explaining fertility transitions. Demography 34(4):443–454
McDonald P (1993) Fertility transition hypotheses. In: Leete R, Alam I (eds) The revolution in Asian fertility: dimensions, causes and implications. Clarendon Press, Oxford, pp 3–14
McDonald P (1994) Families in developing countries: idealised morality and theories of family change. In: Cho J, Yada M (eds) Tradition and change in the Asian family. East-West Center, Honolulu, pp 19–28L
McDonald P (2000a) Gender equity in theories of fertility transition. Popul Dev Rev 26(3):427–439
McDonald P (2000b) Gender equity, social institutions and the future of fertility. J Popul Res 17(1):1–16
McNicoll G (1980) Institutional determinants of fertility change. Popul Dev Rev 6(3):441–462
McNicoll G (1985) The nature of institutional and community effects on demographic behaviour: a discussion. In: Casterline J (ed) The collection and analysis of community data. International Statistical Institute, Voorburg, pp 177–184
McNicoll G (1994) Institutional analysis of fertility. In: Lindahl-Kiessling K, Lanberg H (eds) Population, economic development and the environment. Oxford University press, Oxford, pp 199–299
Montgomery M, Casterline J (1996) Social learning, social influence, and new models of fertility. Popul Dev Rev (Suppl) 22:151–175
Moore R (2007) Family planning in Iran, 1960–79. In: Robinson WC, Ross JA (eds) The global family planning revolution: three decades of population policies and programs. The World Bank, Washington D.C., pp 33–58
Notestein F (1945) Population – the long view. In: Schultz T (ed) Food for the world. University of Chicago Press, Chicago, IL, pp 36–57
Notestein F (1953) Economic problems of population change. In: Proceedings of the eighth international conference of agricultural economists, Oxford University Press, London
Richards A, Waterbury J (1998) A political economy of the Middle East, 2nd edn. Westview Press, Boulder, CO
Robinson WC (1997) The economic theory of fertility over three decades. Popul Stud 51(1):63–74
Robinson WC, Ross JA (eds) (2007) The global family planning revolution: three decades of population policies and programs. The World Bank, Washington D.C
Shadi-Talab J (2005) Iranian women: rising expectations. Critique: Crit Middle East Stud 14(1): 35–55
Szreter S (1993) The idea of demographic transition and the study of fertility change: a critical intellectual history. Popul Dev Rev 19(4):659–701
Thompson W (1929) Population. Am J Sociol 34(6):959–975
Wilson C, Airey P (1999) How can a homeostatic perspective enhance demographic transition theory? Popul Stud 53(2):117–128

Chapter 2
The Social, Economic and Cultural Contexts of Population Policy Changes in Iran

Introduction

Fertility decline in Iran needs to be set within the socio-economic and cultural context of the twentieth century and particularly the post-revolutionary era. This includes the progress of institutional development, particularly in rural areas, legitimization of family planning programs by religious leaders and government officials, the rise of education, and the improvement of health services in rural areas.

This chapter reviews population dynamics, population policy and social changes in Iran during the twentieth century. The aim is to provide the social–institutional context within which the fertility decline occurred over the last three decades.

A Brief History of Population Dynamics

At the beginning of the twentieth century, the population of Iran was estimated to be around 10 million increasing to 13 million by 1933 (Bharier 1968, pp. 274–275). If these population estimates are correct, the rate of growth in the first third of the twentieth century was just 0.8% per annum. Iran's population continued to grow at a slow rate until the late 1940s. This was despite the fact that Iran's traditional pronatalist culture (which emphasized early and universal marriage as a social and religious value) as well as prevailing health and social conditions (high infant mortality and dependence of parents on children as the main source of old-age support) provided an environment for high fertility. During this period, mortality offset the high fertility and kept the rate of population growth at a low level. The first national census of population and housing conducted in 1956 revealed a population of 18.9 million with an average annual growth rate of 1.7% (Maroufi Bozorgi 1967; Amani 1970, 1996; Saraie 1997). Ten years

M.J. Abbasi-Shavazi et al., *The Fertility Transition in Iran: Revolution and Reproduction*,

later, according to the 1966 Census, the Iranian population had risen to about 25.8 million implying an average intercensal growth rate of 3.1% per annum (Bulatao and Richardson 1994; Mirzaie 2005). Thus, in the second third of the twentieth century, Iran moved from a high mortality–high fertility population to one with high fertility and relatively low mortality, fitting the classic demographic transition (See also: Amani 1996; Saraie 1997).

In 1966, Mohammad Reza Shah signed the *Statement on Population of World Leaders* drafted and circulated by John D. Rockefeller and backed by the United States' Government (www.popcouncil.org/mediacenter/popstatement.html). The statement was essentially a commitment to implement family planning programs to bring the high rates of population growth under control. Iran's first family planning program began at this time. After a decade of the family planning program (1967–1976, discussed in the next section), the third national census taken in 1976 revealed a population of 33.7 million and an average annual intercensal growth rate of 2.7%, suggesting modest success of the program. However, following the Islamic revolution and in the context of the Iran–Iraq War, Iran's population once again grew very rapidly. The 1976–1986 average annual growth rate was 3.9% mainly due to the pronatalist approach taken after the Revolution. By 1996, the Iranian population had reached 60 million, a more than six fold increase in a century (Statistical Centre of Iran 1996) but the remarkable fall in the birth rate was well underway following the implementation of the second family planning program as discussed below.

Figures 2.1 and 2.2 show the age pyramids for Iran in 1976, 1986, 1996, 2000, and 2006 providing a visual representation of the changes in the Iranian population over a century. Three observations can be made about these pyramids. First, considerable improvement is evident in the amount of age heaping and digit preference from 1976 to 2000. This is important because this study uses the own-children method of fertility estimation that is reliant upon the accuracy of age reporting in censuses and sample surveys (Chapter 3). Second, the very young age structure of Iran arising from the high fertility during the 1976 and 1986 period is clear in the figures. Since 1990, the huge concentration of the population in the teenage years has presented the government with severe pressures in the supply of education, health and other social needs especially employment. For the purposes of this book, it has almost certainly provided a strong sense of competition in education and employment among the parents of this large generation and among the generation itself. Third, the remarkable decline in births since the mid 1980s is also clearly evident in the 1996 Census, the 2000 IDHS and the 2006 Census age distributions. This is evidence in itself of the timing and extent of fertility decline. By 2006, the very large cohorts born in the 1980s were entering the childbearing ages. This would have produced a huge expansion in births had it not been for the substantial fall in fertility that has occurred in Iran. In the conclusion to the book (Chapter 10), the implications of changing cohort sizes for future births in Iran are discussed.

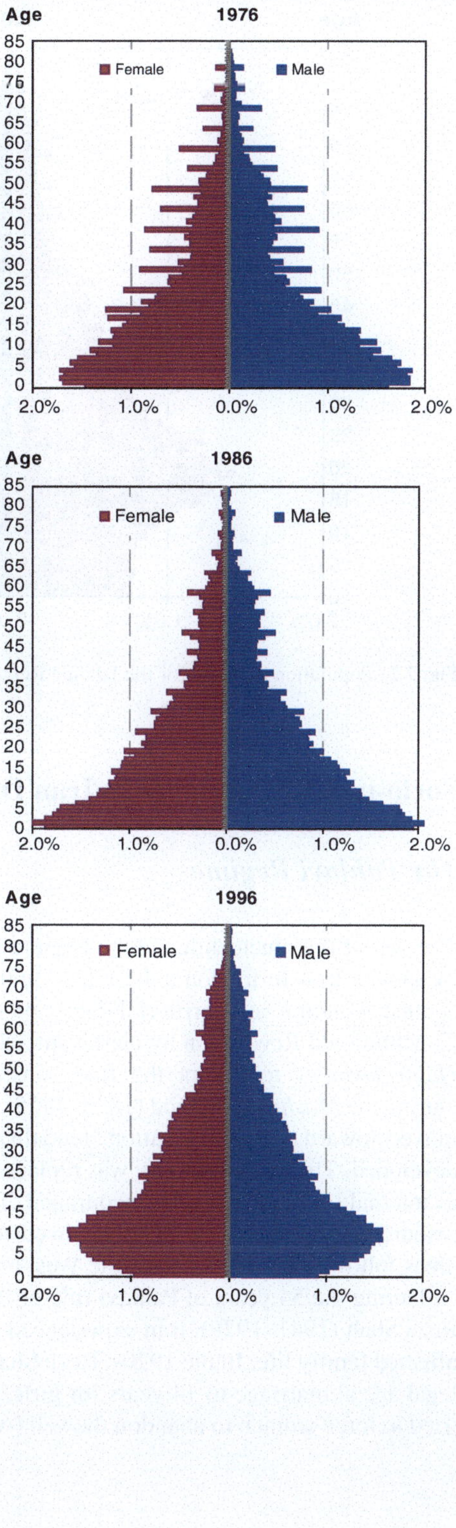

Fig. 2.1 Population pyramids for the Islamic Republic of Iran, 1976, 1986 and 1996 (Statistical Centre of Iran, the 1976, 1986 and 1996 censuses)

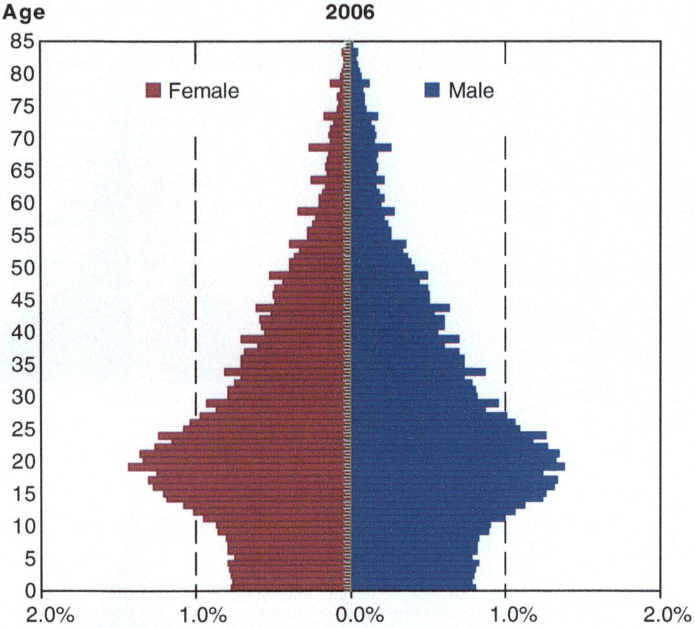

Fig. 2.2 Population pyramid for the Islamic Republic of Iran, 2006 census

Socio-political Changes in Iran During the Twentieth Century

The Pahlavi Regime

The end of the nineteenth and the beginning of the twentieth century were marked by a major transformation in Iran. During the period, 1905–1911, Iranians protested against economic and territorial domination by Britain and Russia which led to the Constitutional Revolution by clerics, merchants, and intellectuals forcing the weak *Qajar Dynasty* to accept the first constitution and Parliament (Wright 2000). During the *Mashrotiat* period (1895–1925), Iran was opened to the West, the society moved towards industrialization, feudalism weakened and a state apparatus was developed. The rural economy was replaced by a cash economy and foreign as well as internal investments were encouraged. This industrial investment needed human resources, and thus rural people moved to cities. Migration from rural to urban areas followed by migration to the West brought about social changes.

During the 54 years of Pahlavi rule of Reza Shah (1925–1941) and Mohammad Reza Shah (1941–1979), Iran experienced major social and economic changes that affected family life. In the 1920s, Reza Shah enacted laws to increase the minimum legal age at marriage to 14 years for girls, passed a compulsory education act, and tried to force women to abandon the veil (*chador* and *hijab*). The Family Protection

Law limited the unilateral right of men to divorce as well as the practice of polygamy without the consent of the first wife. Work opportunities for women were increased but women's employment had risen only to a still-low 14% by 1976. Vatandoost (1985, pp. 107–114) singled out three major initiatives by these monarchs that affected the general status of Iranian women. The first was a 1935 decree by Reza Shah banning the public use by women of the *Chador* (the veil). During his 16 years of absolute rule, Reza Shah took major steps to centralize power and to achieve a degree of westernization and modernization. In his efforts to provide an impression of Iran as a modern nation, he attempted to abolish all visible symbols of traditionalism, such as the veil and the native attire for men, and to replace them with Western dress and headgear. However, there was religious opposition to these measures and, as a result, the policy on the unveiling of women was not rigidly enforced under Md. Reza Shah.

The second major initiative was a decree by Mohammad Reza Shah granting Iranian women the right to vote as well as to run for and hold public office. On 9 January 1963, he outlined a six-point reform program that is known as the *Shah's White Revolution referendum.* The six-point reform program consisted of: (i) land reform, (ii) nationalization of forests, (iii) sale of shares of government-owned industries in order to finance land reform, (iv) profit-sharing with workers in order to prevent the exploitation of labor, (v) formation of literacy corps and (vi) amendments to election laws granting voting rights to women. Sabahi (2002) claims that the White Revolution was promoted by the Kennedy administration as an alternative to a potential red revolution, as a way to combat communist subversion and as a condition of the receipt of U.S. aid. The White Revolution was aimed at propelling Iran to the level of the most modernized countries before the end of the century. However, religious leaders (*ulama*) believed that there were hidden motives behind the Shah's White Revolution. They argued that any initiative by the Shah, who was regarded as pro-United States, could only be self-serving and, in the long run, this would mean a further loss of Iran's independence (Vatandoost 1985, pp. 113–114).

The third initiative of the Pahlavi period was the 1967 legislation entitled the Family Protection Law that granted certain rights to Iranian women by attempting to create legal obstacles to the exercise by men of a unilateral privilege to multiple marriages and to terminating a marriage at will (Vatandoost 1985, p. 107). The law reduced the unilateral right of men to divorce, and polygamy became subject to the consent of the first wife. Women were also given the right to divorce, and the custody of the children after divorce was subject to the agreement of the couple, and, in cases of dispute between the two, the court had the right to make the decision based on the best interests of the children. According to the law, men had to obtain the written permission of the first wife in order to marry a second wife. However, the age at marriage for boys and girls was not changed in the 1967 Family Protection Law (Vatandoost 1985, p. 114). In 1974, the *Majlis* amended the 1967 Family Protection Law. One of the amendments was the increase in age at marriage for girls to 18 and for boys to 20. These amendments were not implemented fully but their symbolic value was very important, indicating that women's rights were officially recognized (Hoodfar 1996, p. 107; Makhlouf Obermeyer 1994, p. 46).

These legal changes may have been successful to the extent that they were initiated in response to the needs of the society in general and women in particular. However, some of the initiatives, including the banning of the veil, received criticism and were resisted by sections of the society and specifically by religious leaders as the changes were regarded as western-oriented and authoritarian. Vatandoost (1985, p. 125) argued that the lack of success of the Pahlavi regimes in changing the status of Iranian women was chiefly due to their equation of social reform with modernization, and modernization with westernization. He noted that Reza Shah was convinced that even Western attire was necessary for social reform and that 'the traditional Islamic belief and institutions were incompatible with a realization of the country's goals, and were therefore expendable.' Similarly, his son did not differentiate between reform and westernization; in his autobiography, he presents the need for westernization as a welcome ordeal.

The 1979 Islamic Revolution

The past three decades of Iran's history have been marked by a series of unprecedented events with immense consequences for the political organization and economic development of the country. The period began with a relatively quick and non-violent popular uprising that started in late 1978 and quickly led to the downfall of the regime that had long been regarded as one of the most stable monarchies of the Middle East.

Almost immediately after the success of the Islamic Revolution, steps were taken to draft a Constitution and have it ratified by public referendum. Shortly after the ratification of the Constitution and the election of its first parliament and president, the Islamic Republic of Iran was subjected to economic blockade by the United States and open military aggression by Iraq. The 8 year war (1980–1988) that ensued was associated with enormous losses in human, economic and material terms. The economic infrastructure, particularly oil production and export facilities, were heavily damaged. As a result, from 1980 to 1988, oil revenue on which the economy depended was reduced to almost one-third of its 1977 value. The decline of the oil revenues and other ravages of the 8 year war soon led to a steady decline in Iran's Gross National Product. The social and human consequences of the war were even more taxing. A large number of villages, towns and cities near the Iraq border were reduced to rubble by enemy fire.

Shortly after the formal end of the war (July 1988), the government of the IRI embarked upon a massive reconstruction program that included two five-year development plans. An explicit emphasis on sustainable human development, social equity, and poverty eradication was a major aim of the First Five-Year Development Plan and maintained its central position in the Second Five-Year Development Plan (Mehryar et al. 1999).

The 1997 landslide election of the reformist president, Mohammad Khatami, was another turning point in the post-revolutionary era, which heralded a democratization period when various political groups formed and the society experienced profound shifts on political issues. Freedom of speech and expression of different values and attitudes became more prevalent and restrictions on peoples' personal and individual behaviour became somewhat more limited. In form, this has been reversed to a large extent with the return of conservatism under the Ahmadinejad presidency but, at the time of writing, changes in the everyday social and economic lives of Iranians had been small. The economy is still weak, education levels continue to rise and family planning continues to thrive. Conservatives and reformers alike perhaps hamstringed by the dualism of government in Iran seem to be wary of radical change.

The Shah's Family Planning Program

The history of the pre-revolutionary family planning program goes back to the establishment of the Department of Health in 1955 to deal with maternal and child health care issues. The first family planning clinic started its activities and services in 1958. In 1962, the government included population issues in the Third Development Plan (1963–1967), and in 1964, a *fatwa* was issued by Sheikh Bahaoddin Mahallati indicating that 'the use of contraceptives is permitted if they are temporary and do not make the woman sterile'. In 1966, a delegation from the Population Council visited Iran to study population issues as well as health and family planning programs. One year later, the Undersecretary of Population and Family Planning was established within the Ministry of Health and the government officially began its family planning activities. The program became active during the Fourth Development Plan (1968–1972) and various health centres at different levels were established during this period. In 1972, the then Director General of the Family Planning Department announced that the objective of the program was to reduce the Crude Birth Rate from 48 to 40 births per 1,000 population, and to accomplish this goal, the program needed to provide family planning services to around 3.6 million women of reproductive age, and prevent around 1 million unwanted births (Kaveh-Firouz and Abbasi-Shavazi 2004).

The Fifth Development Plan (1973–1977) reinforced population policy. The plan aimed to reduce the total fertility rate from an estimated 7.0 in 1972 to 3.0 births per woman in 1992. While much was to happen in between that was not envisaged in 1972, it is ironic that this target level was subsequently reached soon after 1992, about 1995. The other objectives of the program were the implementation of the family planning program as a national strategy with special emphasis on rural areas, the expansion of the health system and family planning services in collaboration with public and private organizations, educating people and families, studying population dynamics, and amendment of laws which were seen to be in opposition to the family planning program. The government had planned to implement a more comprehensive program during the Sixth Development Plan (1978–1982), but the plan could not be implemented due to the 1979 revolution.

The Shah's family planning program was targeted primarily at urban middle class women and was followed by a number of initiatives to improve the status of women, the most important being the introduction of the Family Protection Laws in the late 1960s and 1970s. Although its coverage of the population was somewhat narrow, the program was relatively successful among those that were targeted. The population growth rate declined to 2.7% per annum during the period 1966–1976. Thus, the pre-revolutionary family planning program contributed to a moderate fertility decline and offset the large impact of mortality decline on the population growth rate. It also diffused knowledge of family planning methods and contraceptive use through much of the country. Mirzaie (2005) has observed that the main emphasis of the pre-revolutionary family planning program was on the training of medical and paramedical personnel and the provision of clinic services with a lesser emphasis placed on understanding and solving the cultural, social and economic barriers to fertility control, especially in rural areas. The program, 'like most such programs at the time, stressed the "supply side": the availability of contraception' (Bulatao and Richardson 1994, p. 20). Thus, it could not be as effective and successful as had been planned. However, although the program did not achieve its goals fully during the 1970s, it laid a foundation for the success of the post-revolutionary family planning program.

Suspension of the Family Planning Program

In the early years of the revolution, the pre-revolutionary family planning program was rejected by religious leaders who argued that the program was counter to Islamic values and stemmed from the West. The anti-Shah movement questioned every plan and activity that the regime had implemented during the 1960s and 1970s. As a consequence, the family planning program was suspended shortly after the revolution. Although, the government did not formulate a specific pronatalist policy, several socio-cultural and economic policy changes were made that were effectively pronatalist in nature. First, the office of Under Secretary of Population and Family Planning was abolished, and family planning staff members were moved to other departments of the Ministry of Health. Second, the minimum legal age at marriage, which was increased by the Family Protection Laws, was again reduced to 13 and 15 for girls and boys, respectively. The reduction of age at marriage was considered to be necessary to prevent further moral and social corruption. Religious leaders emphasized marriage and family formation as basic Islamic virtues, and the government was urged to adopt economic policies that would facilitate and encourage early and universal marriage (Hoodfar and Assadpour 2000). Third, the Iraq–Iran war beginning in September 1980 created a pronatalist atmosphere that affected population policies and fertility control in many ways. The creation of a popular *"Twenty Million Man Army"* proposed by Ayatollah Khomeini, the leader of the revolution, was adopted as a national slogan early in the war. It has been argued that the rising casualties of the war may have encouraged many middle-aged couples to produce more children to replace those whose loss they were anticipating (Abbasi-Shavazi et al. 2002; Mehryar 2005).

From the beginning, the war and its consequences gained much of the attention of the revolutionary government. Other social issues including the family planning program did not gain much priority. To provide for the basic needs of the people in a wartime situation, particularly poor people, a universal rationing system was introduced as a means of ensuring equal access to basic necessities. The rationing system included not only basic food items but also locally produced or imported modern consumer goods like television sets, refrigerators, carpets and even cars. These were distributed on a per capita basis and larger families were entitled to a better share of both the basic commodities and highly prized modern consumer items (Abbasi-Shavazi et al. 2002). Thus, the rationing system may have had an indirect impact on peoples' perceptions of the cost and benefits of children. All of these policies were ideological approaches to the fulfilment of the slogans of the revolution on the reduction of inequality in the society.

The impact on population of policies implemented in the early years of the revolution is contested. Ladier-Fouladi (1997, p. 191) has argued that the political and legal resurgence of Islam in these years was not responsible for the higher level of fertility. She suggests that changes in the law, and more specifically the institutionalization of the *Sharia* did not affect demographic developments. On the other hand, while the Islamic government did not implement any explicit policies to increase the population, some of the social and economic changes after the revolution can be considered to be pronatalist in their effect. This applies especially to the suspension of the family planning program. At the same time, as we argue in a later section, the development policies of the government such as the expansion of education and adult literacy, the greatly increased coverage of the health network system and rural development contributed to the strengthening of lower family size ideals in the society.

The Emergence of Post-revolutionary Antinatalist Policy

The demographic consequences of the pronatalist approach after the revolution did not take long to become evident. The 1986 Census indicated that the population of Iran had grown at an average annual rate of 3.9% per year during the 1976–1986 period despite the large losses from the war. The unexpectedly large population size (49.3 million) revealed by the 1986 Census was at first hailed as a "God-sent" gift, but soon became a "wake-up call" for planners (Richards and Waterbury 1998, p. 86). Publication of the 1986 Census results focussed attention on the long-term economic and social implications of the high rates of fertility and population growth. Government officials including those at the Ministry of Health and the Budget and Planning Organization, became very concerned about the consequences of high population growth and its impact on the future of development programs in the country. In an in-depth interview for this book conducted by Abbasi-Shavazi, Masood Roghani Zanjani, the then head of the Budget and Planning Organization and deputy to the then Prime Minister, Mir Hossein Mousavi, said that he had discussed the issue of the consequences of the war and its impact on population and development in Iran with the Cabinet and had argued that measures of caution should be taken with regard to population growth. This initiative had been supported by the then Minister for Health, Alireza Marandi, who was later awarded the 2000 UN Population Award for his contribution to the Iranian health system and to the success of the post-revolutionary family planning program. Cabinet supported the initiative by the narrow margin of one vote.

Behind closed door meetings were held with the religious leaders who were the high ranking policy makers, including Ayatollah Ali Khameme-e, the then President who later became Ayatollah Khomeini's successor as the Official Spiritual Leader of the Revolution and with Ayatollah Hashemi Rafsanjani, the then Parliament Speaker to gain their support for the revival of the family planning program. Officials were advised to take precautionary steps to decrease the negative views that people may have gained from the previous opinions of religious leaders on the Shah's family planning program. Ayatollah Makarem Shirazi, one of the influential clerics in Qom Seminary *[hozah-e elmiyeh]*, in another interview with the first author, mentioned that 'during the early years of the revolution, religious leaders were not convinced about the necessity of the family planning program. However, as it became clear that the large population increase would have a considerable social, psychological, economic and cultural impact on peoples' lives as individuals, and on Iran's population as a nation, then they (religious leaders) provided their support for the family planning program'.

The Plan and Budget Organization, as the national agency responsible for the monitoring and allocation of the government's financial resources, was in a unique position to know the critical state of the war-shattered economy and its fast-dwindling ability to support a large and rapidly increasing population. To raise public support for the idea of population control and family planning, a three- day 'Population and Development' seminar jointly organized by the Ministry of Health and the Planning and Budget Organization was held in Mashhad in September 1988. The recommendations of this seminar explicitly called for the adoption of a national population policy aimed at birth control. At the end of the Mashhad seminar, the Minister of Health and Medical Education, in a press conference, reiterated Imam Khomeini's *fatwa* regarding the legitimacy of contraceptive use by consenting couples, and announced that a family planning program would soon be established. Almost simultaneously, the Prime Minister declared that "birth control" was a "destiny factor" for Iran and invited Iranian women to prevent unwanted pregnancies by seeking help from government-run clinics and rural health houses. To overcome any misconception regarding the legality of birth control, the head of the judiciary system publicly declared that the use of contraceptive methods for preventing unwanted pregnancies was not against Islamic criminal law (Abbasi-Shavazi et al. 2002; Mehryar 2005).

Following the Mashhad seminar, family planning was considered by a group of eminent clergy and religiously-minded physicians attending a seminar on "Islamic Perspectives in Medicine" organized by the Mashhad University of Medical Sciences in February 1989. This was followed by another seminar explicitly dealing with "Islam and Population Policy" which was held in Isfahan in April 1989, and brought together a large number of eminent theologians and politically influential clergy. Most of the recommendations of the Mashhad seminar were taken into consideration in the preparation of the First Five Year Development Plan (FFYDP). The idea and objectives of population control and family planning were given formal legislative endorsement when the FFYDP bill was approved by the Islamic Legislative Assembly (*Majlis*) in 1989. This was 4 years before the eventual enactment of the Family Planning Law of the IRI in 1993. Other details of this fundamental policy reversal and its success in such a short period of time have been elaborated elsewhere (Malekafzali 1992; Hoodfar and Assadpour 2000; Kaveh-Firouz and Abbasi-Shavazi 2004; Mehryar 2005).

The FFYDP also set some relatively modest demographic targets for the newly established family planning program. These included reduction of the total fertility rate of Iranian women from 6.4 in 1986 to 4 by the year 2011 and reduction of the natural rate of growth of the population from 3.2% to 3.05% by the end of the Plan (1993) and to 2.3% by the year 2011. To reach these goals, the coverage of public family planning services was to be extended to 24% of eligible couples by the end of the FFYPD (Plan and Budget Organization 1989, pp. 2–6).

In line with the above-mentioned goals, the Ministry of Health and Medical Education (MOHME) was given the mandate and the resources to provide free family planning services to all married couples, to promote small family size norms and to help individual couples keep their family size at a reasonably low level (2 to 3 children). Several other Ministries as well as the Islamic Republic of Iran Broadcasting Organization were required to closely cooperate with the Ministry of Health in promoting these objectives. A separate Population and Family Planning Directorate was set up within the Ministry of Health in 1991 under the overall supervision of the Deputy Minister for Public Health whose office was also in charge of the primary health care and maternal and child health services.

To further ensure the intersectoral cooperation needed, an interdepartmental Family Limitation Commission was set up by a Cabinet decree passed in September 1990. Headed by the Minister of Health, the Commission was to include the Ministers of Health, Education, Higher Education, Labour and Social Affairs, National Guidance, and Plan and Budget as well as the head of the Civil Registration Organization of the Ministry of Interior. The main functions of the Commission were to "monitor, supervise and coordinate all government policies and activities bearing on the control of the population growth rate, to report on steps taken by member agencies, to make recommendations on the formation of a High Council on Family Planning and its functions and membership, and to review proposals made for changing laws and regulations that may encourage or inhibit population growth". A remarkable feature of this decree is the attention it gave to such "beyond-family-planning" measures as the reduction of infant mortality, facilitation of women's education and employment, and extension of social security and retirement benefits to all parents so that they would not be motivated to produce a large number of children as a source of old-age security and support.

Most of these points were also incorporated into the Family Planning Law that had been prepared in 1989 but was finally ratified by the Parliament in May 1993. This law not only removed almost all economic incentives for high fertility and large families, but also provided the necessary statutory basis for the population control policy and family planning program envisaged as part of the First Five-Year Plan of Development initiated in 1989. The Parliamentary Bill concerning the Second Five-Year Development Plan of the IRI (SFYPD) passed in 1994 also reiterated the IRI government's commitment to population control and family planning (See also: Abbasi-Shavazi et al. 2002, pp. 27–29; Mehryar 2005).

The Impacts of the Post-revolutionary Family Planning Program

As discussed earlier, the pre-revolutionary family planning program did not pay much attention to the socio-cultural and religious context. As a result, the program had not reached its goals a decade later because it had not been well received, particularly in rural areas. From 1966 to 1976, there was a modest fertility decline, but it was restricted to urban areas and may have occurred without the family planning program (Aghajanian and Mehryar 1999; Mirzaie 2005).

In contrast, the family planning program implemented in December 1989 was accepted much more readily. By mobilizing various government organizations and the mass communication network, the program succeeded in diffusing ideas throughout the entire country about the value of small families and about methods of family limitation. This situation was reinforced by the support of religious leaders and high government officials who were convinced that the high population growth rate was having a negative effect on the development of the country in general and on the standard of living in particular. The prior spread of public health services across the country also facilitated the implementation of the program through these services.

Caldwell (1993, p. 307) has argued that religion was an important obstacle to family planning in Pakistan and countries further west in Asia. It was also important at the government and sometimes the personal level among Muslims in Malaysia and Catholics in the Philippines. There have also been religious and ethnic differentials in contraceptive use in other countries. For example, in 2000, the contraceptive prevalence rate was much lower for Malays than for Chinese in wealthier Malaysia (Peng 2002, 2007). However, the support of religious leaders in Iran legitimized the family planning program and the government was able to provide family planning services to people without any religious barriers. This religious legitimization also paved the way for the printing of family planning brochures, the teaching of population education in high schools, the holding of workshops for young couples, and other educational campaigns by the mass media. Commenting on the success of family planning in Iran, Wright (2000, p. 165) wrote that 'the Islamic Republic had been more successful in reaching a wider audience, as compared with the monarchy, because it had won the approval from the clergy, many of whom had called just a few years earlier for the birth of an Islamic generation'. As Aghajanian (1995, p. 3) noted, the most important aspect of Iran's success in family planning is the interest, support and guidance of religious leaders, and this holds implications for other societies with strong religious traditions. Owing to the legitimization of family planning, not only has there been no major religious barrier to the implementation of the family planning program and the use of contraceptives, but also birth control has been advertised as the social and religious duty of couples and individuals.

Irrespective of the merits of the arguments surrounding the rise in fertility in the early 1980s, there is no doubt that birth control has become a central element in the lives of young couples since the late 1980s. The high level of contraceptive use in Iran is an indication of the strength of demand for contraceptives but can also be considered as an indicator of the success of the family planning program in the last decade (See Chapters 6 and 7). The contraceptive prevalence rate (CPR) rose from 37% in 1976 to around 72% in the year 2000. The CPR in rural areas increased from 20% in 1976 to 67% in 2000; the corresponding figures for urban areas are 54% and around 78%, respectively (Mehryar 2005; Hosseini-Chavoshi 2007).

The Context of the Family Planning Program

Hoodfar and Assadpour (2000, p. 20) portray the pre-revolutionary approach to development as "trickle-down theory of economics" because of its concentration on building an urban middle class, while the post-revolutionary approach gave priority to meeting the population's most basic needs, particularly to target the poor and less privileged. The slogans of the revolution also targeted the poor. The Islamic Republic's development policies therefore were focused upon rural development and the expansion of education and health throughout the country, particularly to rural and deprived regions of the country as described in this section.

Expansion of the Health Network System

The health system during the 1940s and 1950s was very sparse and the majority or rural areas did not have access to health services. In the late 1940s and 1950s, a number of targeted health projects including the Malaria Reduction Project were implemented in order to eliminate the main sources of infectious disease. Then, during the 1960s and 1970s, various attempts were made to modernise the country and reduce the inequality between rural and urban areas. Under *the Shah's White Revolution*, the Health Corps [*Sepaheyan-e Behdasht*] and the Literacy Corps [*Sepaheyan-e Danesh*] were employed and sent to rural and deprived areas of the country to improve literacy and health levels. The Shah's regime had also planned to establish a health network system throughout the country. West Azarbaijan Province was selected as the pilot and the aim was to expand the system throughout the country. However, the project was not implemented because of the revolution.

Another initiative directed at improving the health of the deprived regions and rural areas was the employment of foreign medical practitioners from countries such as Bangladesh, the Philippines and Pakistan who were sent to remote areas to provide services to rural people. This plan was continued until the late 1980s.

Two years after the revolution, in 1981, the officials at the Ministry of Health decided to implement the health network system that had been planned by the previous regime. The central aim was to expand the access of people in rural and deprived areas of Iran to primary health care. By 2000, there were around 15,000 health houses [*khanah-e Behdasht*] throughout the country (Mehryar et al. 2005). Each health house covers around 1,500 population in a village and the surrounding satellite villages. Health houses in rural areas follow an integrated health approach. The main functions of a well-established health house include educating the public about health matters, providing family planning and reproductive health services, offering case findings and disease control services, promoting environmental health as well as collecting, recording, storage and periodic reporting of health information and taking an annual census of the population covered by the centre.

Each health house has one or two health officers [*behvars*], one man and one woman, who are appointed by the Department of Health. They usually have high school education but receive 2 years training as a health officer. They also receive on-the-job training from time to time and attend workshops organised by the Department during the year. The training follows an integrated approach and training covers such areas as environment, and maternal and child health care. *Behvars* are usually native to the village and live in the village all the time, and thus, are well known to the people. Because *behvars* know all or most of their clients, they approach them for follow-up treatment or family planning services. The *behvars* is also a channel for referral of people to higher levels of the health system. Due to the establishment of the health network system in the 1980s, health officers initially were young and enthusiastic about their activities, and this contributed to the success of the system in Iran over the last two decades. However, as they have become older and as communications have improved and the demand for health services more complex, reform of their role is on the agenda.

In addition to the village health houses, there are health centers at the district level as well as in urban areas. Health houses are usually supervised by the Rural Health Centres situated in the same rural district. Unlike the activities of health houses in rural areas, the activities of the health centres in urban areas are passive. However, there have been voluntary groups who were trained to approach women in urban areas. While there is a need for reform of the existing health structure in keeping with changed needs and technology, significant reform has been delayed by the unfavourable economic situation (see also: Shadpour 1994, 2001; Mehryar et al. 2005; Salehi-Isfahani et al. 2009).

Until the mid-1980s, the Ministry of Culture and Higher Education was responsible for the higher education system including both medical and non-medical universities. However, in 1985, the Parliament passed a law that put all schools of

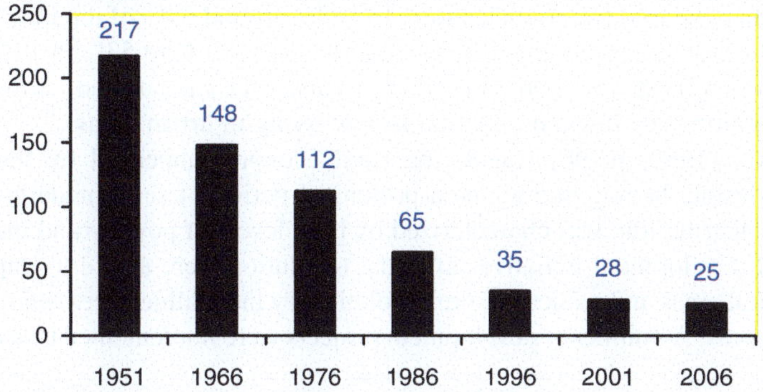

Fig. 2.3 Trend of infant mortality rate in Iran, 1951–2006

medical and paramedical sciences under the direct control of the Ministry of Health and Medical Education. The reason for this was to integrate both health and medical education under one ministry. By the late-1980s, medical universities had trained sufficient doctors and practitioners to enable the government to cease the employment of medical doctors from other countries. Indeed, in the 1990s, an over-supply of medical practitioners emerged and the Ministry of Health and Medical Education along with the Ministry of Employment and Social Affairs made some arrangements for medical doctors to practice in some African and Arab countries.

It is not surprising that the health indicators in post-revolutionary Iran have improved substantially. The establishment of the health network system and its extension to rural and deprived areas of the country has been one of the key factors in reducing infant mortality. The infant mortality rate remained high at about 112 per 1,000 live births in 1976 (Fig. 2.3). This is roughly equivalent to the levels that applied in Western countries around the time of the commencement of their fertility declines. However, the rate in Iran fell sharply to 65 by 1986, 35 in 1996, 28 in 2001 (Mehryar and Tajdini 1998; Mehryar et al. 2005; UNFPA 1998, p. 11; Mirzaie 2005; Abbasi-Shavazi et al. 2005, p. 152) and 25 in 2006. As discussed in Chapter 1, the improvement in child survival may have been a factor in the demand for fewer births and a smaller family size.

Rural Development

Studies have shown that the socio-economic situation in rural areas of Iran before the revolution differed substantially from the situation in urban areas (Shakoori 2001). This led to a large increase in migration from rural areas to urban areas over the past 50 years. The percentage of the population living in rural areas has steadily declined since the mid twentieth century. In 1956, around 69% of the Iran's population lived in rural areas, but this had fallen to 62% by 1966, to 53% in 1976, and to 43% and 39% in 1986 and 1996, respectively (Statistical Centre of Iran, various years). Thus, the majority of Iran's population is now living in urban areas.

As Azkia (1980, p. 96) stated 'the rural economy inherited by the Islamic Republic, despite having undergone a prolonged period of semi-modernist reform and land redistribution, was characterized by high levels of poverty and inequality'. Thus, rural development initiatives after the revolution were aimed to improve the status of rural areas and reduce the pre-revolutionary inequalities between rural areas and urban areas. A number of development projects were implemented to accomplish this goal.

Soon after the revolution, the Construction Crusade Organization or *Jihad-e Sazandegi* was established to revive and develop the cultural, economic and social conditions of rural and deprived regions. The activities of the organization ranged from providing educational and health services to construction of roads and dams, extension of drinking water and electricity networks and distribution of agricultural machinery and equipment. Many rural schools and health centres were built by revolutionary engineers, university students and teachers working voluntarily as *Jihadgar* or Jihad Organization officers during the decade after the revolution. This effort contributed to the establishment of a better and healthier rural environment after the Revolution and made rural areas of Iran significantly different from those of other countries in the region. By 1996, the majority of rural communities had access to electricity, TV, radio and piped water (Table 2.1).

However, Shakoori (2001, p. 91) argued, despite the contribution of *Jihad* in providing services to rural areas, due to the lack of clear planning for development, the programs carried out by *Jihad* have not been fully successful in meeting the basic needs of the rural population. As Azkia (1980, p. 106) has concluded, the post-revolutionary activities failed to eliminate the inequalities between rural and urban areas and did not eliminate rural deprivation. Thus, economic aspirations were raised in rural areas but the reality has fallen short of the expectation.

The Literacy Movement was another organization created after the Revolution. It was aimed at instructing all illiterate persons aged 10 years or more. The organization began its task in 1979 by dispatching volunteer school graduates as teachers to the villages. There were also classes to instruct illiterate employees under 50 years of age working in government offices, factories and workshops.

Post-revolution rural development has many potential implications for the fall of fertility in rural areas of Iran. First, the rise of education increased the cost of children and reduced the benefits of children. Second, the improvements in literacy and education and access to electricity and mass media improved the status of rural women and enlightened their husbands to new ways of thinking. Third, the expansion of the health network system facilitated the fall in infant mortality rates and greatly improved access to family planning services to women. Finally, despite improvements in rural areas, movement to urban areas continued apace with associated implications for lower fertility.

Table 2.1 Selected socio-demographic characteristics of the population, Islamic Republic of Iran, by province

Province	Female literacy (6 years and above)[a] %		IMR		CPR in 1996 [c]		Urban population [b] % 1996	Rural communities with access to: [d] % 1996			
	1986	1996	1986 [a]	1996 [b]	Rural	Urban		Electricity	TV Channel 1	Radio	Piped water
IRAN	52.1	74.2	77.7	34.9	70.1	80.7	61.3	57.5	68.5	87.9	87.2
Ardabil	31.4	64.9	–	45.8	68.7	80.6	48.7	51.5	81.4	88.5	71.5
Azarbaijan E	41.7	68.2	96.7	42.8	76.5	79.9	60.3	56.7	73.9	94.4	81.6
Azarbaijan W	34.3	58.7	103.6	48.1	67.3	78.7	52.7	60.9	80.4	96.0	78.1
Booshehr	50.6	75.2	58.0	43.9	59.1	74.7	53.1	69.1	81.3	91.2	84.6
Charmahal	44.3	70.4	67.2	44.9	67.3	78.5	45.1	55.4	56.9	88.3	92.8
Fars	56.3	77.4	56.2	38.5	68.8	77.7	56.7	50.3	67.0	89.0	94.5
Gilan	58.0	74.6	51.1	31.4	77.6	82.0	46.8	77.4	79.1	95.9	52
Hamadan	43.6	71.3	91.1	46.6	70.3	80.8	41.8	88.7	95.6	96.7	82.7
Hormozgan	41.8	66.6	63.9	45.1	42.5	74.9	48.3	44.3	54.4	78.1	78.7
Ilam	40.0	71.2	78.7	54.1	66.0	75.3	53.2	69.9	74.4	79.6	92.1
Isfahan	62.7	80.9	71.3	32.3	81.8	84.5	74.3	77.1	85.2	91.6	96.6
Kerman	51.5	74.8	75.9	47.1	71.3	80.7	52.9	48.4	56.1	77.3	86.8
Kermanshah	42.8	70.1	74.8	49.4	69.6	77.3	61.8	74.4	75.6	94.9	84.3
Khorasan	46.9	76.8	115.2	51.6	68.8	80.2	56.6	47.0	72.6	91.9	86.9
Khoozestan	48.6	70.0	71.3	41.1	57.7	73.0	62.5	54.8	61.3	84.8	89.4
Kohgilooyeh	39.9	68.3	83.2	58.0	54.2	73.5	39.2	36.8	28.8	88.1	73.9
Kurdistan	23.2	57.4	130.7	63.6	67.3	78.1	52.4	70.6	72.0	97.1	81.8
Lorestan	41.2	68.9	76.4	50.6	61.0	74.9	53.7	57.0	57.6	87.1	84.1
Markazi	51.2	73.9	105.8	41.7	78.0	86.3	57.1	81.7	90.3	92.0	91.5
Mazandaran	54.4	74.6	63.1	42.0	74.8	80.6	45.9	81.7	84.4	96.1	82.5

(continued)

Table 2.1 (continued)

Province	Female literacy (6 years and above)[a] %		IMR		CPR in 1996 [c]		Urban population [b] % 1996	Rural communities with access to: [d] % 1996			
	1986	1996	1986 [a]	1996 [b]	Rural	Urban		Electricity	TV Channel 1	Radio	Piped water
Qom	57.5	77.0	–	37.8	–	–	91.2	80.5	86.1	89.0	98.3
Semnan	63.2	80.8	63.1	37.5	84.6	85.2	68.3	64.5	88.0	93.7	97.4
Sistan & Baluch.	25.3	48.8	83.7	65.4	55.8	68.2	46.1	24.8	37.1	67.8	58.8
Tehran	78.4	85.0	46.3	31.4	79.8	83.9	86.2	79.5	83.7	90.8	97.8
Yazd	61.6	79.8	68.5	37.2	85.3	87.2	75.2	71.2	89.4	96.4	94.6
Zanjan	39.6	67.8	105.9	42.8	69.3	78.6	47.6	75.2	86.3	93.4	86.2

IMR = Infant Mortality Rate; CPR = Contraceptive Prevalence Rate.

[a] Beladi-Mousavi (1997).

[b] Statistical Centre of Iran (1999).

[c] Mehryar et al. (1999).

[d] Mehryar and Tajdini (1998).

The Status of Women in Post-revolutionary Iran

The 1979 Islamic Revolution was in many ways a reaction to some of the initiatives by the Shah that were considered to be western and/or non-Islamic. Soon after the revolution, the Islamic government emphasized domesticity and motherhood as the main roles of women, and reversed some of the policies initiated during the Shah's regime. In regard to marriage, the main legal changes after the Islamic Revolution were the reduction of age at marriage, elimination of the restrictions on polygamy, and the provision of financial support for new couples. Immediately after the Islamic Revolution, the 1967 and 1974 Family Protection Laws were applied only when they were deemed to be consistent with *Sharia* law or *Fatwa*. For example, according to the 1931 Law, the minimum ages at marriage for girls and boys were 15 and 18 respectively, but according to *fatwa*, the minimum age at marriage for girls and boys was 13 and 15, respectively (Bahmani 2000, pp. 46–63).

The *Hijab* (veil) became compulsory and women were required to wear the *chador* and a special form of dress in public areas and offices. Primary, secondary and high schools were segregated for boys and girls. The presence of women in offices was discouraged, and thus, employment opportunities for women became more restricted. As a result, according to the censuses, the female employment rate fell from 14% in 1976 to around 7% in 1986.

However, an egalitarian spirit prevailed in the streets during the period of the Revolution. Both during and after the Revolution, males and females alike joined in the demonstrations, marches, and strikes that culminated in the establishment of the Islamic Republic of Iran. This visible participation of women presented a new image of the female, and women themselves began recognizing their strength in numbers, albeit in the pursuit of conservative causes (Touba 1985, p. 131).

Education is one of the main factors of social change, and operates to promote family change in many ways but especially through improvements in the status of women. Particularly over the last two decades, the level of education has increased rapidly in Iran. Children of all social classes, including the poor, have access to education, and educational differences in the society are continuing to narrow. The literacy rate has increased in both urban and rural areas. Table 2.2 shows the literacy rates for women of prime reproductive ages (15–29) from 1966 to 2006 by rural and urban areas. The literacy rate for women aged 15–19 in urban areas has risen from around 57% in 1966 to around 98% (almost universal) in 2006. The improvement in

Table 2.2 The literacy rate for women aged 15–19 to 25–29, Iran, by rural and urban areas (Statistical Centre of Iran, Various censuses)

Age	1966		1976		1986		1996		2006	
groups	Urban	Rural	Urban	Rural	Urban	Rural	Urban	Rural	Urban	Rural
15–19	57.7	5.4	75.4	19.8	85.8	53.0	96.9	86.4	98.3	93.2
20–24	41.2	2.7	59.4	10.1	75.8	36.5	93.8	77.9	97.9	90.5
25–29	29.5	1.4	49.4	4.9	65.5	22.0	89.5	65.4	96.3	84.1

rural areas has been phenomenal increasing from only 5% in 1966 to 93% in 1996. Similar changes have occurred in the two other age groups, 20–24 and 25–29.

The gender gaps in literacy and education have also narrowed substantially. This has had a considerable impact on the status of women and is, indeed, a central feature of social change in the society. The level of education, particularly for girls, has risen for all social classes (Abbasi-Shavazi et al. 2002, p. 430). The sex ratio of university students has changed in favour of girls. In 1998, around 52% of university candidates who were admitted to government universities were girls. The figure increased to 57% in 1999, and then to around 62% in 2001 (Abdollahyan 2004). Studies suggest that aspirations and expectations of women in post-revolutionary Iran have risen considerably (Mir-Hosseini 2002; Kian-Thiebaut 2002; Shadi-Talab 2005). This has led to the improvement of the status of women at least within the family and women have gained major roles in family decision-making (Azadarmaki and Bahar 2006). Shadi-Talab (2005) noted that 'Iranian girls gradually practice democracy within the family, and patriarchal power is slowly diminishing'. Increased literacy has contributed to women's confidence, and has increased women's perceptions that they have options in many aspects of their lives, particularly women in rural areas who had been constrained by traditional social norms (Hoodfar 1996, p. 35). Girls who stay in education longer are delaying their marriages, and this will affect their fertility decision-making.

Women are increasingly seeing their role as involving work outside the home (Mohseni 2000). Around 73% of women aged 15–49 studied in the Iran Fertility Transition Survey preferred their daughters to continue their education rather than marrying early and this was associated with the view that daughters would need education to find a job in the future. A large majority of women in the survey believed that women should work outside the home to have financial autonomy and also to contribute to the family's income (Abbasi-Shavazi et al. 2003). Another recent action has been the provision of military training to females, and they are now able to become law enforcement personnel, jobs that were not available to them after the revolution. However, these gains in women's education so far have not been associated with much change in their labour force participation, at least as measured by the censuses. There was a noticeable decline (from 12.9% to 8.2%) in the labour force participation rate of women between 1976 and 1986 and only a slight increase to 1996 (9.1%), but the rate for 2006 (16.6%) was almost twice the figure in 1996. The discrepancy in the educational attainment and the labour force participation rate of Iranian women is mainly due to cultural factors that preclude women's employment in such areas as construction, sales, and even food preparation and the hotel industry (Mehryar and Farjadi 2000; Mahmoudian 2006).

Note should also be taken of the publication in recent years of several weekly magazines as well as academic journals that publish articles on women affairs. There was also an improvement in the status of women during the Khatami presidency. Women's participation in the 1997 election was very significant, and Khatami promised to initiate various programs for women's empowerment. For the first time after the revolution, he appointed a woman, Masoumeh Ebtekar as the deputy to the President and Head of the Environment Organization. He also appointed Zahra Shojaie as advisor to the President for women's affairs. Ahmadinejad has also appointed two women to these positions. A number of women representatives have been elected in the parliamentary and rural city council elections. Several non-governmental organizations are also active in women affairs, especially in achieving legal and social changes in favour of women within the government. These women, as noted by Hoodfar (1996, p. 106), have questioned prescribed gender roles and the male interpretation of the proper 'Islamic role' for women, and have encouraged the government to introduce reforms in the areas of marriage, divorce, and education. However, like men, women's engagement in the public sphere applies on both sides of the political spectrum. Conservative women's organizations played an important role in the election of the Ahmadinejad government. This has helped to shore up some of the conservative approaches to women in Iranian society.

Administrative Divisions in Iran: Provinces *(Ostans)*

Until the early 1990s, Iran was administratively divided into 24 provinces (*Ostans*), but the number had increased to 26 by 1996, and to 30 by 2004. Each province is directed by a Governor (*Ostandar*) who is proposed by the Ministry of Interior and approved by the Cabinet. Provinces vary markedly in terms of indices of socio-economic development (Mehryar and Gholipour 1995; Mehryar and Tajdini 1998). Using factor analysis, Kazemi (1999) employed such indicators as the infant mortality rate, the dependency ratio, literacy rates for males and females in both rural and urban areas, the urbanization rate, and male and female life expectancies to rate the levels of development in Iran's provinces in 1986 and 1996. Provinces were given a score of 1 (very low), 2 (low), 3 (medium), 4 (high), and 5 (very high) in terms of their level of development. Sistan-Baluchistan, Kohgiloyeh-Boyerahmad, Ilam, West Azarbaijan and Kurdistan were ranked as low and very low, while Tehran, Semnan, Gilan, Mazandaran, Isfahan and Qom were among the high and very highly developed provinces in both 1986 and 1996. As a centralized society, there is also a pronounced geographical development pattern in Iran. Provinces at the borders of the country tend to be more underdeveloped while those in the central areas and particularly those close to the capital, Tehran, are well developed (Table 2.1). In Chapter 3, we consider fertility trends at the provincial level and examine their association with stages of development.

Iran is also a multilingual and multi-ethnic society. The most important ethnic groups are Arab, Baluchi, Kurd, Lore, Persian, Turk, and Turkmen. Three provinces in the northwest contain Turkish communities and two provinces in the west contain Kurdish communities. In the southern part of Iran, three provinces on the Persian Gulf contain a mixture of Arabs and Persians. Baluchi live in the Province of Sistan-Baluchistan located in the South Eastern part of Iran, while Persians populate the central plateau of Iran (Fig. 2.4). Around 99.5% of the population is Muslim, the vast majority of whom (around 92%) belong to the Shiite sect of Islam;

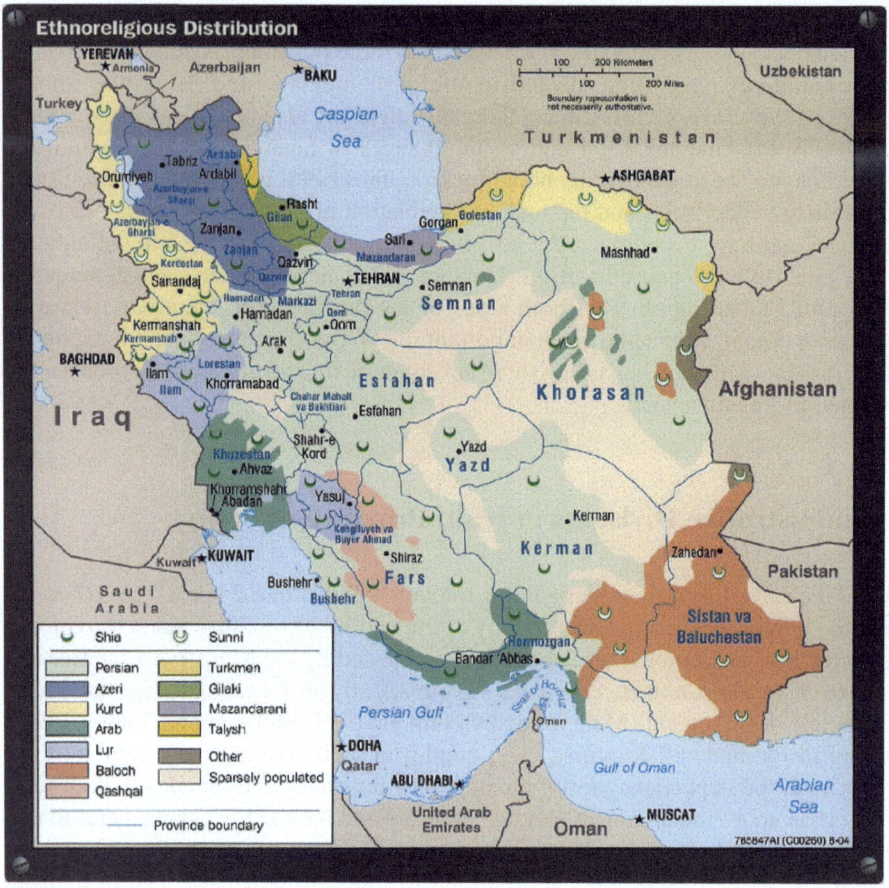

Fig. 2.4 Map of Iran: Ethno-religious distribution (University of Texas Libraries, Perry-Castañeda Library, Map Collection: http://www.lib.utexas.edu/maps/middle_east_and_asia/iran_ethnoreligious_distribution_2004.jpg

and only 8% are Sunni. There are close associations between province of residence, ethnicity and sect of Islam that make it difficult to examine the separate effects of each of these factors upon fertility. In effect, they coalesce into what can be more broadly described as cultural variations.

Conclusion and Discussion

For most of its history since the late 1960s, Iran has had an active family planning program. Initially, this program was a manifestation of the Pahlavi regime's endeavour to display Iran as a modern, enlightened country in the western mode. This endeavour also included changes in marriage laws to protect the rights of women and attempts to reduce the prominence of the veil and to promote women's employment outside the family circle. The impact of this campaign was much more prominent in some of the large urban areas than it was outside these areas. In rural areas, traditional ways largely continued, education levels remained low and access to health services was poor. However, Iran had taken the first steps towards population control and, among predominantly Muslim countries, along with Indonesia, Iran played a leading role in the implementation by government of a family planning program.

Following the Islamic Revolution, family planning activities were curtailed and poverty alleviation programs were set in place that could have had pronatalist effects. The conduct of the war with Iraq may also have had pronatalist effects as families sought to replace their members who had been killed in the war. It appears that fertility rates rose in this period and a large generation of children was born.

Faced with the results of the 1986 Census, those who held to the idea that national and family development would be curtailed by excessive numbers of children were able to have a major political impact. They were able to convince religious and community leaders that population growth could not continue at that rate without producing major negative consequences for economic development. The Islamic Government moved to re-invigorate the family planning program and its implementation proved to be more effective than had been the case under the Shah's regime. Most important religious leaders actively supported the new program. The advantages of family planning were preached in the mosques. This was in striking contrast to Pakistan (Hakim 2005), and also to Malaysia (Peng 2002, 2007). The spread of the national public health system to all regions of the country and to village level meant the program could be delivered effectively and efficiently to most women in the country. And women across the country were more receptive to the idea of family planning because of the greatly improved levels of literacy. Women's education levels and the quality of the health system have continued to improve over the past 30 years further cementing the direction of change.

On the other hand, over the past 30 years, successive Iranian governments have achieved very little success in relation to economic reform. Even today, the economy is characterised by protection and the propping up of inefficient state enterprises. The wealth generated by oil revenue has not been transformed into the development of a vibrant economy and economic growth has remained low. Economic sanctions are a contributor to this situation. The combination of poor economic results with rising education levels and rising economic aspirations, besides creating some frustration among the Iranian people, has led families to seek ways in which their economic outcomes can be improved. With the employment of women still largely restricted, one of their options has been reduction of the number of children that they have.

This provides a broad background to the social and economic context of the decline of fertility in Iran in the past two decades. In the following chapters, we examine this fertility decline in considerable demographic detail. This detail may shed some light on the extent to which the fall in fertility can be seen as part of a longer term process dating back 40 years or more, a process that was temporarily slowed down by the Islamic revolution, or whether it can be attributed primarily to changes in the past 20 years. Irrespective of the answer to this question, there can be no doubt that fertility has continued to fall rapidly in a country widely regarded as religiously conservative. This defies the conventional wisdom of the past and requires explanation.

References

Abbasi-Shavazi MJ, Mehryar A, Jones G, McDonald P (2002) Revolution, war and modernization: population policy and fertility change in Iran. J Popul Res 19(1):25–46

Abbasi-Shavazi MJ, McDonald P, Hosseini Chavoshi M (2003) Changes in family, fertility behavior and attitudes in Iran. Working Paper in Demography No. 88. Australian National University, Australia

Abbasi-Shavazi MJ, Hosseini-Chavoshi M, Koosheshi M, Naghavi M (2005) Trends and emerging issues of health and mortality in the Islamic Republic of Iran. In: United Nations, Economic and Social Commission for Asia and the Pacific (ed) Emerging issues of health in mortality in the Asian and Pacific region. United Nations, New York, pp 147–160

Abdollahyan H (2004) The generations gap in contemporary Iran. J Welt Trends 44:78–85

Aghajanian A (1995) A new direction in population policy and family planning in the Islamic Republic of Iran. Asia-Pacific Popul J 10(1):3–20

Aghajanian A, Mehryar A (1999) Fertility transition in the Islamic Republic of Iran: 1967–1996. Asia-Pacific Popul J 14(1):21–42

Amani M (1996) An attempt on historical outlook of the trends of births and death rates and study of the stage of demographic transition in Iran [Persian]. J Popul 13–14:71–83

Amani M (1970) Births and fertility in Iran (Persian). University of Tehran, Division of Population Research, Institute for Social Studies and Research, Tehran

Azadarmaki T, Bahar M (2006) Families in Iran: changes, challenges and future. J Com Fam Stud, 37(4):589–607

Azkia M (1980) The effects of rural development programmes on the Iranian peasantry between 1962–1978. D. Phil. Dissertation, Aberdeen University, Aberdeen

Bahmani E (2000) Confrontation of family with modernism with emphasis on legal aspects (Persian). MA thesis in Sociology, University of Tehran, Tehran

Beladi-Mousavi S (1997) Female socio-economic indicators in the Islamic Republic of Iran (Persian), Office of Women's Affairs, President Office, Tehran

Bharier J (1968) A note on the population of Iran, 1900–1966. Popul Stud 22(2):273–279

Bulatao RA, Richardson G (1994) Fertility and family planning in Iran. Middle East and North Africa Discussion Paper Series, No. 13. World Bank, Washington, DC

Caldwell J (1993) The Asian fertility revolution: its implications for transition theories. In: Leete R, Alam I (eds) The revolution in Asian fertility: dimensions, causes, and implications. Clarendon Press, Oxford, pp 299–316

Hakim A (2005) Fertility trends and their determinants in Pakistan. In: Jones GW, Karim M (eds) Islam, the state and population. Hurst, London, pp 233–253

Hoodfar H (1996) Barganing with fundamentalism: women and the politics of population control in Iran. Reprod Health Matters 8(November):30–40

Hoodfar H, Assadpour S (2000) The politics of population policy in the Islamic Republic of Iran. Stud Fam Plann 31(1):19–34

Hosseini-Chavoshi M (2007) Fertility regulation in Iran: An analysis of trends, levels and correlates. Ph.D. thesis in Demography, Australian Demographic and Social Research Institute, The Australian National University, Canberra

Kaveh-Firouz Z, Abbasi-Shavazi M-J (2004) Population policy change and its impact on fertility in Iran (Persian). Proceedings of the first conference of the Population Association of Iran. Population Association of Iran, Tehran

Kazemi R (1999) Socio-economic determinants of fertility in Iran, (Persian). MA thesis in Demography, Faculty of Social Sciences, The University of Tehran, Tehran

Kian-Thiebaut A (2002) Women and the making of civil society in post-Islamist Iran. In: Hooglund E (ed) Twenty years of Islamic revolution: political and social transition in Iran since 1979. Syracuse University Press, Syracuse, pp 56–73

Ladier-Fouladi M (1997) The fertility transition in Iran. Popul: Engl Sel 9:191–214

Mahmoudian H (2006) Socio-demographic factors affecting women's labour force participation in Iran. Critique: Crit Middle Eastern Stud 15(3):233–248

Makhlouf Obermeyer C (1994) Reproductive choice in Islam: gender and state in Iran and Tunisia. Stud Fam Plann 25(1):41–51

Malekafzali H (1992) Population and family planning programs in the Islamic Republic of Iran [Persian]. Nabz J Contin Educ 2:3–7

Maroufi Bozorgi N (1967) Population projection for Iran, 1956–1976. In: Proceedings of the World Population Conference, Belgrade, 30 August–10 September 1965, vol 3. Selected papers and summaries: projections, measurement of population trends. United Nations Department of Economic and Social Affairs, New York, pp 19–22

Mehryar A (2005) Shi'ite teachings, pragmatism and fertility change in Iran. In Jones G, Karim M (eds) Islam, the state and population. Hurst and Co, London, pp 118–156

Mehryar A, Farjadi G (2000) Labour force participation of women in Iran. Institute for Research on Planning and Development, Tehran

Mehryar AH, Gholipour R (1995) Provincial differences in fertility in Iran, 1976–1991. Institute for Research on Planning and Development, Tehran

Mehryar A, Farjadi G, Abbasi H (1999) Government spending on basic social services and its share of the GDP and total government budget in the Islamic Republic of Iran, 1971–1999. Institute for Research on Planning and Development and United Nations Children's Fund (UNICEF), Tehran

Mehryar A, Tajdini F (1998) Population and development in the Islamic Republic of Iran: a review of the main findings of the 1996 Census and other sources of data. Working Paper. Institute for Research on Planning and development, Tehran

Mehryar A, Aghajanian A, Ahmad-Nia S, Mirzaie M, Naghavi M (2005) Primary health care system, narrowing of rural-urban gap in health indicators, and rural poverty reduction: the experience of Iran. Paper presented at the IUSSP conference, Tours, France, 18–23 July 2005

Mir-Hosseini Z (2002) Religious modernists and the "woman question". In: Hooglund E (ed) Twenty years of Islamic revolution: political and social transition in Iran since 1979. Syracuse University Press, Syracuse, pp 25–33

Mirzaie M (2005) Swings in fertility limitations in Iran. Critique: Crit Middle Eastern Stud 14(1):25–33

Mohseni M (2000) Study of knowledge, attitudes, and socio-cultural behaviours in Iran. Tehran

Peng Tey Nai (2007) The family planning program in Peninsular Malaysia. In: Robinson WC, Ross JA (eds) The global family planning revolution: three decades of population policies and programs. World Bank, Washington, DC, pp 257–276

Peng Tey Nai (2002) Social, economic and ethnic fertility differentials in Peninsular Malaysia. Paper presented at the IUSSP Conference on Southeast Asia's Population in a Changing Asian Context, held at the Siam City Hotel, Bangkok, Thailand, 10–13 June 2002

Plan and Budget Organization (1989) The first plan of economic, social and cultural development of the Islamic Republic of Iran (1989–1993) bill, Appendix 1 [In Persian]. Plan and Budget Organization Press, Tehran

Richards A, Waterbury J (1998) A political economy of the Middle East. Westview Press, Boulder, CO

Sabahi SF (2002) The literacy corps in Pahlavi Iran (1963–1979): ISIM Newsletter 10:19

Salehi-Isfahani D, Abbasi-Shavazi MJ, Hosseini-Chavoshi M (2009) Family planning and rural fertility decline in Iran: a study in program evaluation. Paper presented at the 2009 Meeting of the American Population Association, Detroit, MI, 30 April to 2 May 2009

Saraie H (1997) Demographic transition of Iran: a preliminary report [Persian]. J Soc Sci 9:1–18

Shadi-Talab J (2005) Iranian women: rising expectations. Critique: Crit Middle Eastern Stud 14(1):35–55

Shadpour K (2001) The integrated approach to primary health care in the Islamic Republic of Iran. In: Mehryar A (ed) Proceeding of the first international workshop on integrated approach to reproductive health and family planning in the Islamic Republic of Iran, 31 April – 13 May 2000, Isfahan. Institute for Research and Development Planning, Tehran, pp 177–187

Shadpour K (1994) The primary health care experience in Iran. UNICEF, Tehran

Shakoori A (2001) The state and rural development in post-revolutionary Iran. Palgrave, New York and Hampshire, UK

Statistical Centre of Iran. Various years. 1976, 1986 and 1996 Censuses. Statistical Centre of Iran, Tehran

Statistical Centre of Iran (1996) Iran statistical yearbook. Statistical Centre of Iran, Tehran

Statistical Centre of Iran (1996) Iran population data sheet. Statistical Centre of Iran, Tehran

Touba JR (1985) Effects of the Islamic revolution on women and the family in Iran. In: Fathi A (ed) Women and the family in Iran. E. J. Brill, Leiden, pp 131–147

United Nations Population Fund (UNFPA) (1998) Country report on population, reproductive health and family planning program in the Islamic Republic of Iran. Ministry of Health and Medical Education, Tehran

University of Texas Libraries, Perry-Castañeda Library, Map Collection. http://www.lib.utexas.edu/maps/middle_east_and_asia/iran_ethnoreligious_distribution_2004.jpg

Vatandoost GR (1985) The status of Iranian women during the Pahlavi regime. In: Fathi A (ed) Women and the family in Iran. E. J. Brill, Leiden, pp 107–130

Wright R (2000) The last great revolution: turmoil and transformation in Iran. Alfred A. Knopf, New York

Chapter 3
National and Provincial Level Fertility Trends in Iran, 1972–2006*

Introduction

This chapter documents the changes in fertility in Iran since the 1970s. Own-children data from the 1986, 1996 and 2006 Censuses as well as the 2000 Iran Demographic and Health Survey (IDHS) enable analysis of single-year fluctuations of fertility over the last three decades. The chapter describes the levels, trends and patterns of fertility in Iran by rural and urban areas during the period 1972–2006. Then, provincial-level fertility trends and patterns are examined for both rural and urban areas. Next, attention is given to the attainment of below-replacement level fertility in various provinces of Iran.

The results show that Iran experienced a modest decline in fertility during the 1970s followed by a rise in fertility between 1976 and 1984. The rise was, however, short lived. The total fertility rate began to decline from 1985 and has declined sharply since 1988 dropping from 5.5 in 1988 to the replacement level in 2000 and to 1.9 in 2006. The decline has been observed in all provinces and urban and rural areas of the country despite varying levels of socio-economic development. Several provinces and urban as well as rural areas of the country have experienced below-replacement level fertility.

Data and Method

The 1986, 1996 and 2006 Censuses and the 2000 Iran Demographic and Health Survey (IDHS) are used to provide estimates of fertility levels and trends over the last three decades based on the own-children method. The own-children method is an indirect technique that uses the reverse-survival procedure to estimate fertility measures for the years prior to a census or household survey (Cho et al. 1986, p. 1). Based on the information on the household record, children under the age of 15 are

---

*Other versions of this chapter were published as Abbasi-Shavazi and McDonald 2005, 2006.

M.J. Abbasi-Shavazi et al., *The Fertility Transition in Iran: Revolution and Reproduction*,

matched to women aged 15–64 in the same household, with the assumption that the women are the mothers of the children enumerated in the same household. This provides a table of all matched children by their own age and the age of their mothers at the time of the enumeration. An adjustment is made to include children where a match to a mother cannot be made. This is done on the assumption that the mothers of unmatched children have the same age distribution as the mothers of the matched children. A life table appropriate to the population is then used to reverse survive the children back over each of the 15 years proceeding the census or survey to obtain the number of births by age of mother in previous years. The numbers of women at each age at the enumeration are also reverse survived using the life table to obtain estimates of the numbers of women at each age in the population in each of the previous 15 years. Age-specific fertility rates and total fertility rates are then calculated for each year by dividing the number of reverse-survived births by the number of reverse-survived women. The details and the application of the technique have been elaborated elsewhere (Cho 1973; Cho et al. 1986; Grabill and Cho 1965; Jain 1989; Rindfuss 1977; Retherford et al. 1979).

Several reasons justify the use of the own-children method in Iran (Abbasi-Shavazi 1999, 2001a). The first reason is the incompleteness of vital registration data. Vital registration in Iran was not complete during the 1970s and 1980s but the level of completeness has improved since the 1990s (Ladier-Fouladi 1997). Second, there have been substantial improvements in census coverage and age reporting in recent censuses in Iran (Saraie 1995; Leete and Alam 1997; Mirzaie et al. 1996, Keshtkar 2000). The improvement in age reporting in recent censuses is attributed to the rising levels of education as well as to the fact that the interviewers registered age on the basis of respondents' identity cards. This contributed greatly to the accuracy of age reporting at the 1996 Census. Single-year age distributions of the population of Iran in the 1976, 1986, 1996 Censuses and the IDHS were evaluated in an earlier paper (Abbasi-Shavazi 2001a). There were some signs of age heaping and digit preference at the 1976 Census, but progressively less so at the 1986 and 1996 Censuses. This conclusion applied to the national level as well as to the province level (except for the few less developed provinces of Sistan and Baluchestan, Ilam and Hormozgan). An assessment of the own-children estimates using the 2006 Census revealed similar results (Abbasi-Shavazi et al. 2008). Third, more than 95% of children under 15 live with their natural mothers in Iran. Fourth, given the fluctuating trend of fertility over the last two decades, and particularly with the sharp decline in fertility in Iran in recent years, unlike other indirect methods of fertility estimation, the own-children method allows estimation of current fertility for a range of years prior to an enumeration. Accordingly, using the 1986, 1996, and 2006 Censuses as well as the 2000 Iran Demographic Health Survey (IDHS), time trends and fluctuations in fertility can be measured for the last three decades.

Estimates of fertility obtained through the own-children method can be affected by age misreporting and under-enumeration. Careful analysis of the results showed that the rates for the single years, 1972, 1973, 1974, 1985 and 1986 based on the 1986 Census, are slightly under estimated. A comparison of own-children fertility estimates with the results obtained from other sources for the early 1970s yields mixed results. Based on several assumptions and adjustments,[1] Ladier-Fouladi (1997) used birth registration data to estimate the level of fertility from 1966 to 1993. She estimated that the TFR declined from around 7.9 in 1966 to 7.2 in 1976, around one child higher than the own-children estimates. Mirzaie (2005) using census data estimated that the TFR declined from 7.0 in 1966 to 6.3 in 1976. Using birth history data from the Iran Fertility Survey, Aghajanian et al. (1992, Table 5) calculated that the TFR in the 1973–1977 period was 6.4. Finally, using data on age specific marital fertility rates from the Population Growth Estimation Survey (Aghajanian et al. 1992) and age-specific proportions married from the 1976 Census, we have calculated the TFR to be 5.8 for the years, 1973–1976.

The own-children method estimates presented in this paper for the early 1970s tend to be on the low end of this range of estimates but the Ladier-Fouladi estimates are very much higher than all of the other estimates. Without further work upon the reasons for the discrepancy between estimates based on adjusted registration data, survey data and census data, it is presently not possible to provide a definitive view of Iranian fertility in the 1970s. More confidence can be attached to estimates in the 1980s and 1990s. Ladier-Fouladi's results for the 1980s and 1990s are more-or-less similar to the results obtained from the own-children method. Certainly the differences in the own children estimates for the years 1982 and 1983 derived from the 1986 and 1996 Censuses (Table 3.2) suggest that the own-children estimates for the period 1972–1974 based on the 1986 census must be regarded as being too low. This is may be a consequence of the somewhat higher proportions of older children (ages 12–14) that do not live with their natural mother (Table 3.1). Overall, however, the percentages of non-own children were very low in all the data sets used.

The results of the own-children method are not sensitive to the level of mortality (Cho et al. 1986, pp. 45–46). However, the results may be biased by migration (Cho et al. 1986, p. 6). Given the increasing trend of rural–urban migration in Iran during

[1] Ladier-Fouladi's (1997) estimates of fertility using birth registration data for the period 1966 to 1993 are based on the following assumptions and adjustments. First, the coverage of births occurring during the 1970s and 1980s was assumed to be incomplete. The author set out to correct the under-registration of births largely on the assumption that births not registered in the year of occurrence were registered in a later year except for those that may have died in the interim. The author had access to births registered in the year of occurrence and after the year of occurrence only for 2 years, 1984 and 1987. The extent of late registrations was estimated as the arithmetic mean for these 2 years and then this value was assumed to apply to the entire period 1966–1993. The distribution of births registered late was available by the age groups of the child at the time of the registration: age groups 1–4, 5–9 and 10+. These were broken up into single years using an assumed distribution and this assumed distribution was also applied across the entire period. The number of registered births was available for 1992 and 1993 but information on the births registered late were not available for these years. Specific adjustments were made for late birth registrations during these 2 years. Because there may have been deaths of children not registered in the year of birth, Coale and Demeny model life tables were used to convert the estimated numbers of late registrations by age into births the appropriate number of years before the late registration. The numbers of women at each age in each year were estimated based on the 1966, 1976 and 1986 censuses using the forward survival method. Finally, since the distribution of births by mother's age group was not available, Syrian fertility data was used to calculate the number of births by mother's age group for Iran.

Table 3.1 Percentages of children matched to their mothers in the household, Iran, 1986, 1996 and 2006 Censuses and the IDHS 2000

		1986 Census		1996 Census		2006 Census		IDHS 2000	
Age	Total	Matched	Unmatched	Matched	Unmatched	Matched	Unmatched	Matched	Unmatched
0	100	97.5	2.5	97.7	2.3	98.3	1.7	98.3	1.7
1	100	97.9	2.1	97.9	2.1	98.5	1.5	98.2	1.8
2	100	98.0	2.0	97.9	2.1	98.1	1.9	98.0	2.0
3	100	98.0	2.0	97.9	2.1	98.2	1.8	98.1	1.9
4	100	98.0	2.0	97.9	2.1	98.1	1.9	97.8	2.2
5	100	97.9	2.1	97.9	2.1	97.9	2.1	97.3	2.7
6	100	97.7	2.3	97.8	2.2	97.5	2.5	97.2	2.8
7	100	97.5	2.5	97.8	2.2	97.3	2.7	97.0	3.0
8	100	97.4	2.6	97.6	2.4	97.3	2.7	97.0	3.0
9	100	97.2	2.8	97.4	2.6	97.0	3.0	96.8	3.2
10	100	96.8	3.2	97.3	2.7	96.7	3.3	96.8	3.2
11	100	96.6	3.4	97.0	3.0	96.6	3.4	96.4	3.6
12	100	96.0	4.0	96.7	3.3	96.1	3.9	96.0	4.0
13	100	95.7	4.3	96.4	3.6	95.7	4.3	95.7	4.3
14	100	94.8	5.2	96.0	4.0	94.9	5.1	94.7	5.3
Total	100	97.1	2.9	97.4	2.6	97.1	2.9	96.8	3.2

the 1980s, the own-children estimates for urban areas of migrant-receiving provinces may be slightly over-estimated because children enumerated in an urban area at the census may have been born in a rural area. Having considered the effects of age reporting, mortality, migration and matching of children to their mothers on the own-children fertility estimates, Abbasi-Shavazi (1999, 2001a, b) concluded that the method produced satisfactorily reliable fertility estimates for Iran from the 1980s onward. Finally, from 1981 onwards, total fertility rates calculated from synthetic parity progression ratios obtained from the 2000 IDHS were very similar year by year to those obtained by the own-children method (Hosseini-Chavoshi et al. 2006).

Fertility Levels, Trends and Age Specific Patterns: A Detailed Description

This section presents total fertility rates (TFRs) and age specific fertility rates (ASFRs) for Iran from 1972 to 2006. TFR is the average number of children that a group of women would have throughout their lifetimes if they experienced the age specific fertility rates that applied in the given calendar year. It has been claimed that the highest TFR ever recorded was nine children per woman for the Hutterites, a religious sect in the United States (Eaton and Mayer 1953). However, in this study, we observe rates as high as nine or more children per woman in a few provinces of Iran in the early 1980s (see Fig. 3.4). The lowest TFR for a country has been recorded as 0.95 for China Macao ASR (Population Division of the Department of

Economic and Social Affairs of the United Nations Secretariat 2009). However, a level of 0.6 births per woman has been observed for the city of Shanghai in China, The ASFR is the number of children per woman (or 1,000 women) in an age group in a given calendar year. The rate of childbearing is lowest in the youngest and oldest age groups, and fertility reaches a maximum in the central childbearing years. The causes of this variation are the age patterns deriving from the proximate determinants of fertility (Bongaarts and Potter 1983, p. 12), as discussed in Chapter 1. For example, the marriage pattern is of major importance in explaining the shape of the age specific fertility curve because the proportion married varies substantially with age. This proportion is lowest in age group 15–19, and this explains why fertility is low in this age group. At older ages, 40 and over, the level of a woman's fecundity falls sharply and this is why age specific fertility is low at these ages. In this section, we examine the trend of fertility (both level and pattern) from 1972 to 2006 for Iran by rural and urban areas and for provinces.

National Trends: Total Fertility Rates: 1972–2006

The fertility transition in Iran has passed through different phases over the last three decades. As mentioned earlier, the first Iranian family planning program was implemented by the Pahlavi regime in 1966. However, the changes in fertility during the late 1960s and early 1970s appear to have been small. TFR decreased from above 7.0 in 1966 (Amani 1970, 1996; Ladier-Fouladi 1997; Mirzaie 2005) to around 6.5 in 1976 (Padidar-Nia 1977, pp. 133–136; Mirzaie 2005).[2] However, due to socio-political changes as well as the revolutionary protests during the years preceding the 1979 Islamic Revolution, like many other government activities, the family planning program became inactive during the years 1977 to 1979. The own-children estimates show that fertility rose again to 7.0 by 1980. Studies (Hosseini-Chavoshi et al. 2006; Salehi-Isfahani and Tandon 2000, and Chapter 6) have shown that the timing of childbearing shifted towards an earlier pattern of childbearing during the early years of the 1980s and this moved the level of fertility upward.

Despite this, the high fertility regime was short lived and fertility started to decline by the mid-1980s. TFR declined from 7.0 in 1980 to around 6.3 in 1986, and further to around 5.6 in 1988 (the estimated figure based on the 1986 Census was 5.5 as compared with 5.8 based on the IDHS). The decline of fertility was slow

[2] The level of TFR for 1966 varied between 7.9 (Ladier-Fouladi 1997), 7.7 (Amani 1970, 1996) and 7.2 (Mirzaie 2005), while that of the 1976 ranged from 7.2 (Ladier-Fouladi 1997), 6.6 (Padidar-Nia 1977), 6.3 (Mirzaie 2005) and 6.1 (own-children estimates). Padidar-Nia (1977, pp. 133–136) estimated that total fertility in Iran was 6.6 in 1974 (8.1 for rural and 4.5 for urban women). He argued that the large rural population, with high illiteracy and poor access to medical facilities, exposed Iran to conditions resulting in very high fertility, and thus, the fertility had been approximately unchanged during two decades – 1956 and 1974. The TFR for Iran in 1974 has also been reported as 6.0 (UNFPA 1998, p. 11).

until the government population policy was reversed and a new family planning program was officially inaugurated in 1989. TFR fell sharply from that time dropping from around 5.6 in 1988 to around 2.8 in 1996, a decline of 50% in 8 years (Table 3.2 and Fig. 3.1). The low level of fertility in Iran was confirmed by the results of the Population Growth Estimation Survey (PGES) conducted by the Statistical Centre of Iran in 1998 (Statistical Center of Iran 1999) and the 2000 Iran Demographic and Health Survey (IDHS). The own-children estimates of fertility for Iran based on the 2006 Census show that the TFR had reached replacement level (2.1) in 2000, and declined further to 1.9 by 2006.

Fertility trends in Iran over the past three decades, and particularly the sharp decline in the 1990s, are interesting and deserve due attention for the following reasons. First, while other scholars have noted the rise and fall of Iranian fertility after the 1979 revolution (Aghajanian 1991, 1995; Aghajanian and Mehryar 1999; Mehryar and Gholipour 1995a; Saraie 1997; Mirzaie 2005), what has not been observed is the relative stability of the trend in the years before the revolution. This suggests that the fertility decline that commenced with the introduction of the family planning program in 1966 had lost its momentum by the end of the 1970s. Second, although the fertility decline accelerated with the reinstatement of the family planning program in 1989, the decline had commenced from 1985 onwards. Third, the very sharp decline of fertility in Iran as an Islamic country is remarkable, particularly considering the socio-political context in Iran in the 1980s as described earlier.

As noted, early evidence of the spectacular decline of fertility in Iran in the late 1980s and early 1990s was greeted with incredulity by many overseas observers as well as some demographers inside Iran (Abbasi-Shavazi et al. 2002). The Five Year Development Plan in the late 1980s targeted a decline in TFR to 2.3 by 2010 and the family planning program was developed around this target. In reality, this target was achieved a decade earlier but, in 1993, Zanjani (1993) had argued that fertility would decline to only 3.85 by the period, 2016–2021. He argued at the time that even this target might not be achieved given the fact that the experience of other countries in Asia such as India, Pakistan and Bangladesh where family planning programs had been implemented earlier was that fertility had declined only slowly. He also pointed out that the family planning program in Iran was not coercive and it might not be as effective as had been planned.

This was also true for the projections made by the Population Division of the United Nations in the 1990s. In the UN population projections, revised every 2 years, the assumed TFR for the 1995–2000 period in Iran was as follows: in the 1990 projections, 4.30; in the 1992 projections, 5.40; in the 1994 projections, 4.52; in the 1996 projections, 4.77; in the 1998 projections, 2.80. Hence, it was not until the 1998 projections that the Population Division accepted the reality of Iran's fertility decline. By this time, the age distribution of the 1996 Census had made it obvious that fertility had fallen much faster than had previously been believed. The 2000 UN projections provided three variants for the future of fertility for the period 2000 to 2050. According to the high, medium and low variants, by 2005–2009, TFR in Iran would decline to 2.60, 2.32 and 1.98, respectively. The corresponding figures for the period 2010–2014 would be 2.60, 2.10 and 1.60, respectively.

Table 3.2 Own-children estimates of total fertility rates, Iran, 1972–2006 (All age-specific and total fertility rates at national, rural–urban, and provincial levels in this chapter were calculated using the own-children method applied to the 1986, 1996 and 2006 Censuses, and the 2000 Iran Demographic and Health Survey. Only figures for urban and rural areas at the national level during 1972–1986 are from Nourollahi 2000)

	Total				Urban				Rural			
	1986	1996	2006	2000 IDHS	1986	1996	2006	2000 IDHS	1986	1996	2006	2000 IDHS
1972	5.9				5.1				6.7			
1973	5.9				5.0				6.9			
1974	6.0				5.0				7.3			
1975	5.7				4.8				6.9			
1976	6.1				4.9				7.4			
1977	6.1				5.0				7.3			
1978	6.2				5.0				7.5			
1979	6.6				5.3				8.1			
1980	7.0				5.8				8.4			
1981	6.8				5.7				8.0			
1982	6.7	6.1			5.7	5.5			7.9	6.9		
1983	6.8	6.3			5.7	5.7			8.1	7.3		
1984	7.0	6.6			5.8	6.0			8.4	7.7		
1985	6.3	6.4			5.3	5.7			7.5	7.6		
1986	6.2	6.2		6.5	4.9	5.4		6.0	6.5	7.8		7.1
1987		5.8		6.1		4.9		5.5		7.2		6.9
1988		5.5		5.8		4.7		5.1		7.1		6.6
1989		5.3		5.9		4.5		5.1		6.8		6.6
1990		5.3		5.5		4.2		4.7		6.4		6.4
1991		4.9		5.1		3.7		4.3		6.1		6.0
1992		4.3	3.9	4.5		3.3	3.6	3.8		5.3	4.4	5.3
1993		3.8	3.6	4.1		2.9	3.2	3.3		4.8	4.1	4.9
1994		3.4	3.2	3.6		2.6	2.9	3.0		4.2	3.7	4.4
1995		2.9	2.8	3.2		2.3	2.5	2.6		3.4	3.2	3.8
1996		2.5	2.8	2.8		2.0	2.5	2.3		2.9	3.2	3.4

(continued)

Table 3.2 (continued)

	Total				Urban				Rural			
	1986	1996	2006	2000 IDHS	1986	1996	2006	2000 IDHS	1986	1996	2006	2000 IDHS
1997			2.4	2.6			2.2	2.2			2.8	3.0
1998			2.3	2.4			2.1	2.1			2.5	2.7
1999			2.2	2.3			2.1	2.0			2.5	2.5
2000			2.1	2.2			2.0	2.0			2.2	2.4
2001			2.1				1.9				2.3	
2002			2.0				1.9				2.2	
2003			1.9				1.8				2.1	
2004			1.9				1.8				2.1	
2005			1.8				1.7				2.0	
2006			1.9				1.7				2.1	

Figures for the 3 years preceding the 1986 Census are lower than the corresponding rates based on the 1996 Census and this may be due to underreporting of children under 2 in the 1986 Census. The rates for the period 1986 and 1996 based on the IDHS are slightly higher than those from the 1996 Census. There are several possible explanations of these small differences including non-response, assumptions made about mortality levels in the past, small differences in the time references of the different measures and under-enumeration. The 1986, 1996 and 2006 Censuses as well as the IDHS were conducted during October–November. Thus the rates for single years refer to 12-month periods prior to the enumeration. For example, the rate for 1980 refers to November 1979–October 1980.

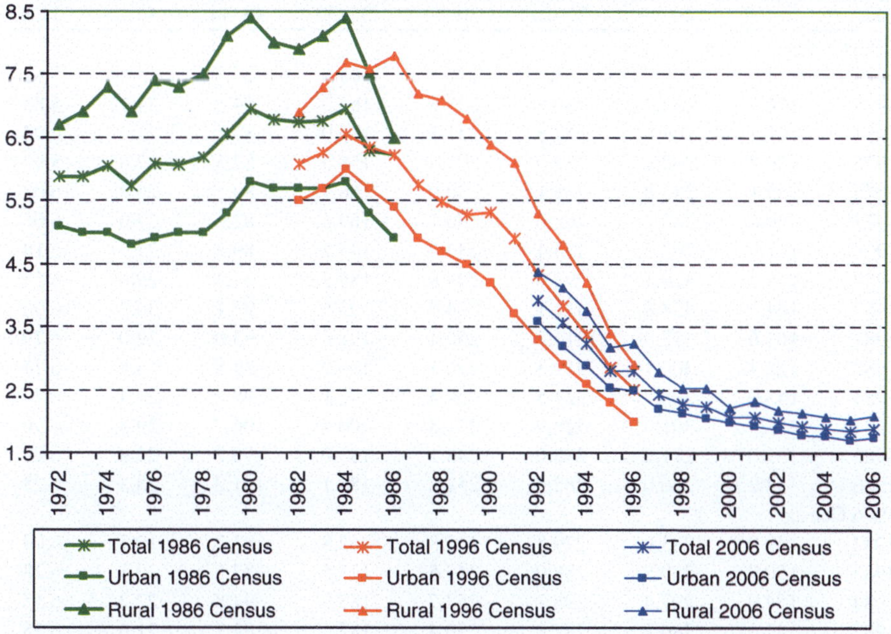

Fig. 3.1 Own-children estimates of total fertility rates for Iran by urban and rural areas, 1972–2006 (see Table 3.2)

Clearly, prior to the 1996 Census, while some earlier evidence was available, demographers were unwilling to conclude that the fall in TFR in Iran was so rapid. In addition, many commentators in the West were unaware of the demographic and social changes inside Iran. Iran was seen only as a conservative Islamic society resistant to many aspects of social change, especially matters affecting women's lives such as family planning.

National Trends: Age-Specific Fertility Rates, 1972–2006

The own-children estimates of ASFRs for Iran for single years during 1972 to 2006 based on the 1986, 1996 and 2006 Censuses as well as the 2000 IDHS are presented in Table 3.3.

As shown in the table, in 1976, the highest age-specific fertility rate was recorded for age group 20–24 (283 per 1,000 women) followed by age groups 25–29 (268 per 1,000 women) and 30–34 (231 per 1,000 women). This age pattern remained in place in 1980 although fertility had risen overall. From 1976 and 1980, rises in fertility were evident for all age groups. However, during the first half of the 1980s, although the TFR remained high and nearly constant, the age pattern shifted towards later childbearing and the peak of childbearing occurred in age group 25–29.

Table 3.3 Own-children estimates of the age specific fertility rates for Iran, 1972 to 2006, 1986, 1996, 2006 Censuses (see Table 3.2)

Year	15–19	20–24	25–29	30–34	35–39	40–44	45–49	TFR
1986 Census								
1972	154.0	259.7	261.7	225.3	164.6	84.1	24.9	5.87
1973	154.4	262.3	260.8	225.8	164.0	84.5	24.1	5.88
1974	161.2	268.8	267.3	231.3	167.9	87.5	25.9	6.04
1975	156.2	262.1	237.0	201.8	158.3	82.5	22.6	5.60
1976	153.1	282.8	268.1	230.9	166.7	89.1	26.4	6.08
1977	140.6	288.7	268.6	230.1	169.6	87.6	27.0	6.06
1978	141.9	292.7	275.4	234.2	175.2	89.3	27.7	6.18
1979	148.3	310.1	292.9	249.8	185.8	94.4	29.6	6.55
1980	164.3	328.8	311.1	264.9	195.6	97.1	30.3	6.96
1981	163.6	312.9	313.2	256.4	191.0	93.0	29.0	6.79
1982	158.4	300.1	319.3	256.1	190.2	95.8	28.8	6.74
1983	155.0	298.7	321.5	260.5	192.1	98.9	28.3	6.77
1984	153.3	301.6	328.9	271.8	200.4	106.7	29.5	6.96
1985	135.0	271.2	298.0	248.1	183.0	98.7	25.9	6.29
1986	132.2	266.0	282.5	252.2	185.1	101.2	28.3	6.23
1996 Census								
1982	149.9	283.9	279.3	235.8	167.8	83.7	19.3	6.09
1983	150.7	289.8	288.0	245.5	175.5	87.5	20.1	6.28
1984	154.0	297.4	298.1	257.7	185.9	94.8	22.2	6.55
1985	147.0	286.7	287.8	250.4	182.4	94.7	21.6	6.35
1986	142.6	277.2	279.5	244.1	183.1	96.1	24.0	6.23
1987	125.8	252.0	257.7	225.1	170.4	87.5	33.6	5.76
1988	115.1	240.9	249.5	219.0	165.1	85.3	22.7	5.48
1989	106.3	232.0	240.8	210.9	159.7	82.2	22.5	5.27
1990	105.1	236.2	244.2	213.5	160.5	83.1	22.9	5.32
1991	101.5	226.1	224.9	191.5	140.5	74.8	22.0	4.90
1992	90.5	207.9	202.8	166.9	117.8	61.8	18.4	4.33
1993	78.4	190.5	184.1	147.0	99.8	50.8	15.6	3.83
1994	68.7	174.4	168.3	127.8	83.3	41.4	13.6	3.38
1995	56.6	153.2	149.3	107.8	66.3	31.3	10.4	2.87
1996	45.3	135.2	136.4	96.2	56.6	25.5	9.1	2.52
2006 Census								
1992	88.8	187.5	186.2	149.5	104.3	50.6	14.4	3.9
1993	77.3	180.6	167.2	137.7	91.0	47.0	11.9	3.6
1994	69.6	165.9	162.6	120.3	78.5	38.5	9.8	3.2
1995	59.0	149.8	143.2	104.4	63.8	29.9	8.1	2.8
1996	56.7	147.0	149.7	105.3	62.6	28.4	8.4	2.8
1997	47.9	132.8	131.5	90.8	51.7	23.1	7.1	2.4
1998	45.2	123.8	127.4	89.4	49.4	18.1	5.0	2.3
1999	41.7	118.0	125.5	90.7	48.8	18.9	4.7	2.2
2000	36.3	110.0	121.3	84.3	43.0	17.2	4.3	2.1
2001	38.1	110.0	120.2	85.7	42.0	16.7	4.5	2.1
2002	35.8	102.9	115.4	86.3	40.7	14.6	4.2	2.0
2003	34.8	99.6	112.3	83.3	40.6	13.4	3.5	1.9
2004	32.7	91.0	112.3	84.0	40.7	13.8	3.8	1.9
2005	32.6	93.7	105.0	80.7	41.8	11.9	3.1	1.8
2006	31.3	92.7	108.6	84.7	42.9	13.4	3.5	1.9

The falls in fertility at younger ages were matched by rises at older ages. Thus, Iranian women had a relatively early childbearing pattern in the first year of the revolution consistent with the pronatalist ideology adopted by the government. This behaviour did not last long however and as age at first marriage increased, fertility shifted to a relatively later childbearing pattern. This result is confirmed by an application of the synthetic parity progression ratio method to the Iran Demographic and Health Survey (Hosseini-Chavoshi et al. 2006, see Chapter 4).

The results show a decline in fertility from 1986 to 1990, particularly in the young age groups, 20–24, and 25–29 in absolute terms. Age specific fertility rates in age groups 25–29 and 30–34 were also lower in 1990 than those in 1986. However, there was a remarkable fall in fertility in all age groups during the 1990–1996 period partly due to the revival and successful implementation of the family planning program during this period. Age specific fertility rates continued to fall from 1996 to 2006, although the rate of decline was slower as there was less scope for further decline during this period. There was also an indication of a further shift towards delayed childbearing during the last period.

The steep fertility decline in all age groups between the periods suggests that simultaneously young couples were starting their childbearing later, married women were spacing their births further apart and older women were stopping their childbearing. The simultaneity of these behaviours explains the very sharp fall in total fertility that has occurred in Iran since the late 1980s. This is examined in more detail in Chapter 4.

Figure 3.2 plots the age-specific fertility rates as a percentage of the rates observed in 1975. This is consistent with our results regarding the rise and fall of

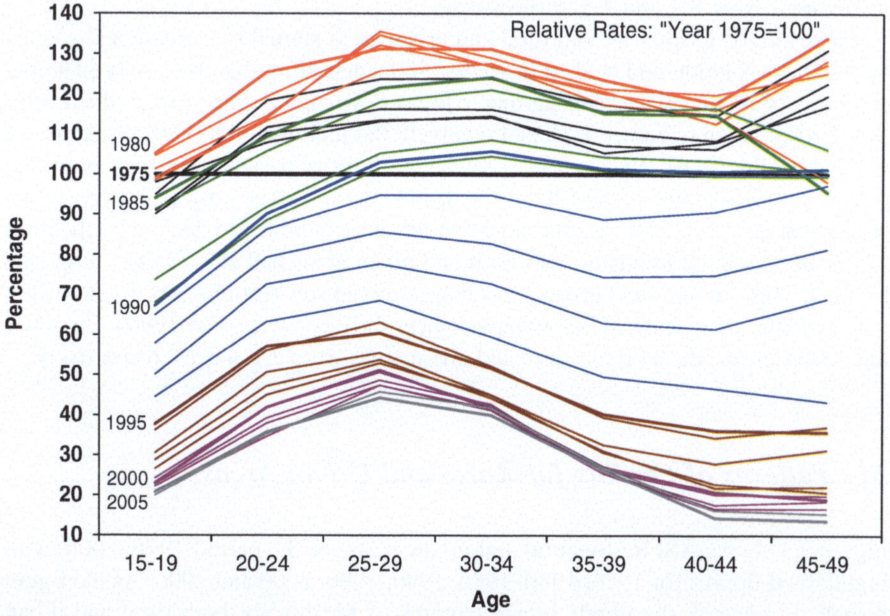

Fig. 3.2 Relative change of age specific fertility rates for Iran, 1975–2006 (see Table 3.3)

fertility in pre- and post-revolutionary Iran. ASFRs increased in all age groups between 1975 and 1980, but there were proportionately larger increases in the mid- and old ages of childbearing. By 1990, the rates in the middle and higher ages of childbearing were close to the 1975 level, but there had been large declines at younger ages. The largest percentage differences between 1975 and 2006 are found at the beginning and end of the reproductive years, resulting in a concentration of childbearing in the central age groups. This compression of the fertility patterns at low levels of overall fertility may have been caused by a rising age at marriage and by a relatively high prevalence and effectiveness of fertility control practised by older women. We return to this in more detail in Chapters 5–7.

Total Fertility Rates for Rural and Urban Areas, 1972–2006

Trends in TFR for rural and urban areas of Iran from 1972 to 2006 are shown in Fig. 3.1. The figure shows fertility according to the place of residence of the woman *at the time of the data collection not at the time of the birth*. Given that urbanisation has been very rapid in Iran over this period, many of the births to women residing in urban areas at the time of the data collection would have occurred in rural areas. As depicted, fertility rates were much higher in rural areas than in urban areas during the 1970s. This is consistent with the findings of other studies (Aghajanian et al. 1992; Koosheshi 1994; Agha 1985; Mehryar and Gholipour 1995a; Mirzaie 2005). Padidar-Nia (1977) had estimated that, in 1974, total fertility rates in rural and urban areas were 8.1 and 4.5, respectively.

Interestingly, fertility in both rural and urban areas started to increase a few years before the revolution and peaked in 1979–1980, suggesting that the family planning delivery system may have been starting to break down in the years prior to the revolution. Fertility then remained high and relatively flat until the mid-1980s. There was a gradual decline from 1986 to 1989, before the fertility transition in both rural and urban areas accelerated in the 1990s. The decline in rural areas was much steeper than in urban areas. The IDHS results show that fertility continued to decline by the mid-1990s, although the trends in both rural and urban areas had slowed. The large gap between TFRs in rural and urban areas has narrowed substantially. The total fertility rate in urban areas reached below replacement fertility by the late 1990s. Based on the 2006 Census, the TFRs in rural and urban areas were 2.1 and 1.7 respectively.

Age Patterns of Fertility for Rural and Urban Areas

Figure 3.3 shows ASFRs for rural and urban areas for the period 1976–2006, with highlighted figures for 1976, 1980, 1986, 1990, 1996, 2000 and 2006. As the figure reveals, in general, the trends in age patterns of fertility for both rural and urban areas during the period were similar to the national level: large declines for all age

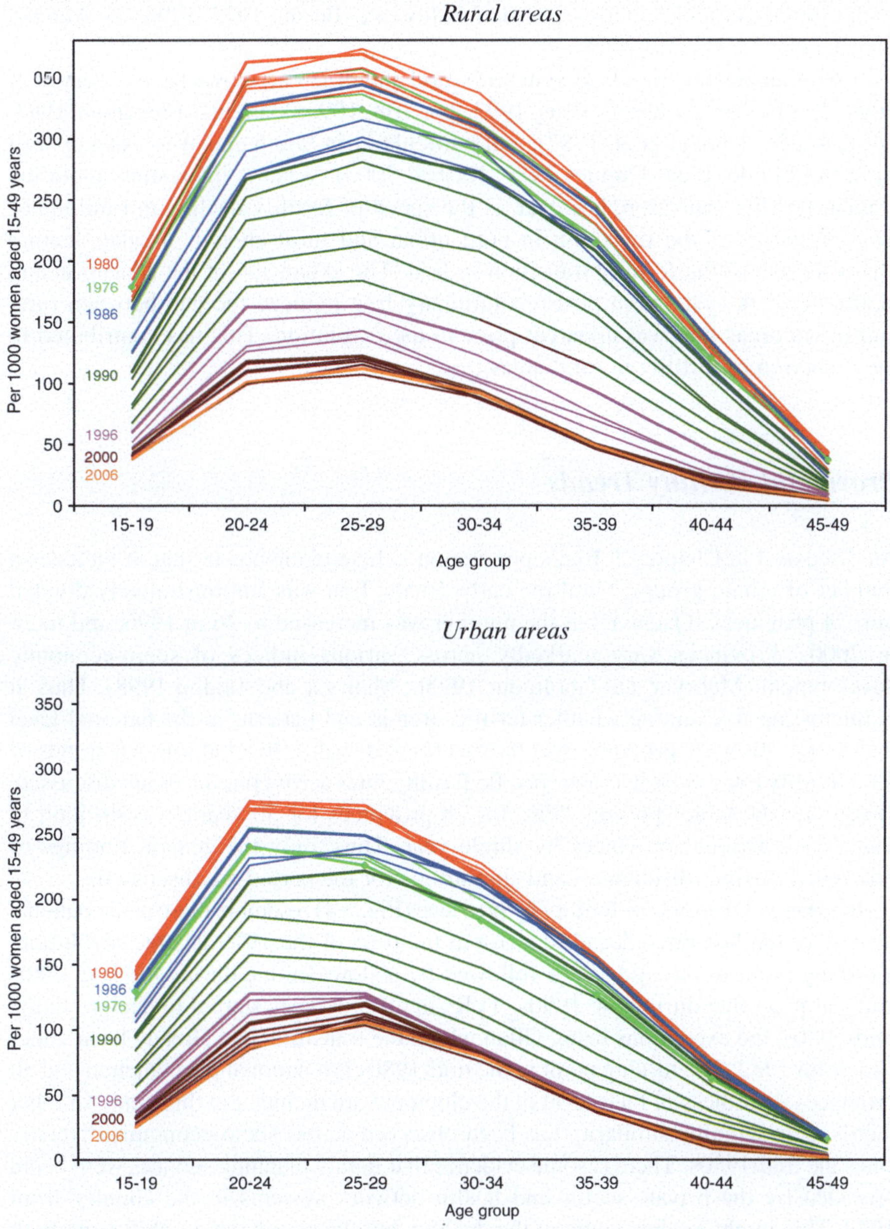

Fig. 3.3 Trends of age-specific fertility rates for rural and urban areas, Iran, 1972–2006

groups with the largest declines being in the young age groups. By the end of the period, rates in rural areas were still falling at all ages, but the falls in urban areas had begun to slow down, especially at the older ages. Consequently, as with the TFR, the gaps between rural and urban areas had narrowed considerably by the end of the 1990s (for tables of age-specific fertility rates during 1972–1996, see Abbasi-Shavazi and McDonald 2005).

Simultaneous fertility decline in both rural and urban areas has been observed in other developing countries (Peng 1993, pp. 108–109; Coale and Freedman 1993, pp. 224–226; Knodel et al. 1987), and particularly in South and West Asia as well as in the Middle East (Fargues 1989; Rashad 2000). What is interesting about the Iranian fertility transition, however, is the speed of fertility decline in rural areas. The similarity of the transition in both urban and rural areas is another feature characteristic of the fertility transition in Iran. The expansion of the education and health network systems in post-revolutionary Iran reduced the gap between rural and urban areas that was apparent prior to the revolution. This has contributed to the reduction of fertility in rural areas.

Provincial Fertility Trends

As discussed in Chapter 2, Iran's population is heterogeneous in that in includes a number of ethnic groups. Until the early 1990s, Iran was administratively divided into 24 provinces (Ostans), but the number was increased to 26 in 1996, and to 28 in 2000.[3] Provinces vary markedly across various indices of socio-economic development (Mehryar and Gholipour 1995b; Mehryar and Tajdini 1998). Thus, it is interesting to examine whether fertility trends and patterns at the national level differ from those by province over the last three decades. In what follows, trends of total fertility rates as well as age specific fertility rates across provinces are discussed. Given that the tables present TFRs for 28 provinces for 30 years, it is difficult to focus on individual provinces by single year. Thus, only the general findings of provincial-fertility differences and similarities for the period are discussed.

In general, the trends of fertility by province (Fig. 3.4) resemble those at the national level over the last three decades; a rise at the time of the 1979 Islamic revolution, a turning point in the mid-1980s followed by a slow decline during the late 1980s and sharp decline during the 1990s. TFRs in all provinces started to decline in the mid-1980s, the exceptions being Gilan where the transition had already been under way from 1982. The turning point in the mid-1980s is a national phenomenon and all provinces regardless of their level of development are included in this trend. In other words, demographic similarity has been observed across socio-economic diversity since the mid-1980s. There is some evidence that family planning services were being provided by the private sector and health network systems in the country from 1984. This might explain some of the decline, but the simultaneous shift from high fertility in 1984 in all provinces needs to be explained. It is also notable that fertility in all provinces declined even before the start of family planning program in 1989.

[3] The number of provinces increased to 30 in 2004 but the focus on this paper is on fertility trends in the provinces included in the 1986 and 1996 Censuses and the 2000 IDHS.

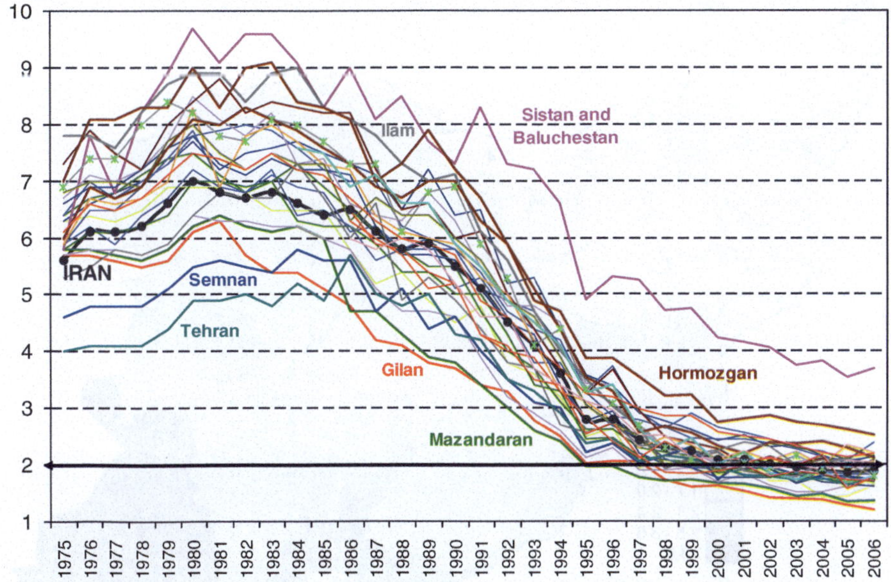

Fig. 3.4 Trends in the total fertility rate by province, Iran, 1972–2006 (see Table 3.2)

Similar to the national trends, a sharp fall in fertility rates was observed in most provinces from 1989 onwards. The speed of the decline since 1989 is remarkable and corresponds in time with the revival of the family planning program in 1989 and the associated endorsements of the program by prominent people in the country (Chapter 2).

In addition, there were marked differences across provinces during the 1970s. A comparison of TFRs for provinces with those for the national average showed that women from most provinces displayed higher fertility, while only a few provinces had lower fertility than the national average in the 1970s and 1980s. However, due to the remarkable downward trend in fertility of most provinces since the late 1980s, provincial levels of fertility have converged to the national level by the end of the period and the provincial fertility gaps during the 1970s and 1980s have now been narrowed substantially (see also Abbasi-Shavazi 2000a, 2002a,b; Abbasi-Shavazi et al. 2007). Figure 3.5, indicates that in 2006, five provinces had TFRs between 1.20 and 1.6, 13 provinces had TFRs between 1.7 and 2.0, while 12 provinces had TFRs between 2.1 and 2.4. Hormozgan province was in the category of TFR between 2.5 and 3.5 with a TFR of 2.5. Sistan-Baluchistan stood out from other provinces with clearly the highest fertility from 1980 onwards (a startling 9.5 children per woman in the early 1980s), and the fertility decline there has continued to lag well behind the rest of the county. Only Sistan and Baluchestan province had a fertility rate in 2006 that was above three (3.7) children per woman.

Studies have shown that the level of fertility in Pakistan's Baluchistan where people of the same ethnicity (Baluchi) are living is higher than other provinces of

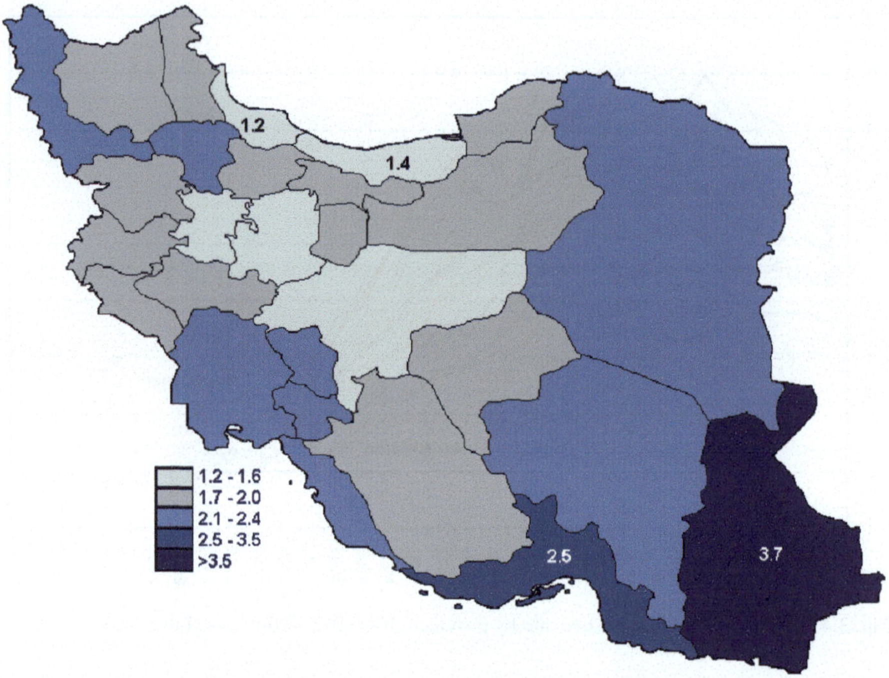

Fig. 3.5 Provincial map of total fertility rate in Iran, 2006

Pakistan (Arnold and Sultan 1992). In 1990/91, the TFR in Pakistan's Baluchistan was estimated by one study to be 5.8 (Arnold and Sultan 1992, p. 41) while, in another study, it was reported to be 7.1 in 1996/97 (Hakim 2001, p. 612). However, the level of fertility in Iran's Sistan and Baluchistan has sharply declined from around 7.5 in 1990 to around 5.5 in 1996, and further to around 4.3 by 2000 and 3.7 by 2006. The high fertility in provinces with the same ethnicity in the two countries of Iran and Pakistan, and the sharp fertility decline in Iran's Sistan and Baluchistan calls for further investigation. Cross-country studies of the fertility of Kurds and Turks in Turkey, Iraq and Iran would also be desirable as they would shed light on the relationship between ethnicity, sect of religion and fertility (see Abbasi-Shavazi and Sadeghi 2006).

Tehran, Gilan and Semnan have displayed considerably lower fertility than the national average and all other provinces. Our analysis showed that Tehran City had the lowest fertility followed by Gilan, Mazandaran, Markazi, Isfahan and Hamadan provinces while on the other hand, Sistan and Baluchistan province displayed the highest fertility followed by Hormozgan, South and North Khorasan, and Kerman as compared with all other provinces in 2006. The very low fertility experienced by Tehran City (1.4 in 2000) and Gilan province (1.2 in 2006) from the early 1990s onwards is an indication of the possibility of very low fertility (below 1.50) being reached in Iran and particularly in urban areas in the future.

To summarise, despite fertility variations across provinces during the period of the study, remarkable downward trends were clearly visible in all provinces. Despite the similarity in fertility trends, there are some differences among provinces. Those provinces with very high fertility declined sharply from eight children per woman in the 1970s to around three to four children per woman in 1996. The speed of the decline in such low-fertility provinces as Gilan, Mazandaran, Isfahan, Tehran, Semnan, Tehran and Yazd was less than that of the high-fertility provinces. The gap between the fertility of provinces with high fertility and the national average has narrowed substantially (Fig. 3.4). As discussed, fertility decline and changes in reproductive patterns have become widespread in provinces of Iran since the mid-1980s.

Fertility Differentials by Province: Age Specific Fertility Rates, 1972–2006

Figure 3.6 shows age specific fertility rates for all provinces during the periods 1975–1977, 1978–1980, 1985–1987, 1988–1990, 1992–1994, and 1998–2000. These figures provide a clear trend and understanding of the unique fertility transition across Iran before and after the Islamic revolution.

The first point to be made is that the general shape of the age specific fertility curves is very similar across provinces. Also, overtime, the fertility pattern changed in broadly the same way across provinces. Between 1975–1977 and 1978–1980, fertility rose in all provinces although the magnitude of the increase varied substantially among the provinces. The rise for such low fertility provinces as Gilan, Mazandaran and Isfahan was not significant, while such provinces as Booshehr, Ilam, West Azarbaijan, Kermanshah, Khouzistan, Khorasan, and Sistan and Baluchistan, characterised by a low level of development, experienced a considerable increase during the early years of the revolution. The increases in fertility were concentrated more at the peak ages of childbearing, 20–34 years.

In the 10-year period, 1978–1980 to 1988–1990, in the high fertility provinces, the rates at all ages tended to fall back to what they had been in 1975–1977. On the other hand, the falls at each age were much more marked in this period for the low fertility provinces: Gilan, Markazi, Isfahan, and Mazandaran. The falls in these low fertility provinces were concentrated in the peak ages of fertility, 20–34 years, rather than in the older ages, although falls are also evident for age group 15–19 in these provinces in this period.

In the next period, 1988–1990 to 1992–1994, large falls were evident in almost all provinces with more of a concentration at the older ages, as would be expected with the recommencement of the family planning program. In the final period, 1992–1994 to 1998–2000, fertility at all ages continued to fall but this time with more emphasis on the two youngest age groups, 15–19 and 20–24. By the final period, age group 25–29 had been established as the peak age for fertility in almost all provinces. By the late 1990s, most provinces displayed relatively similar age patterns of fertility.

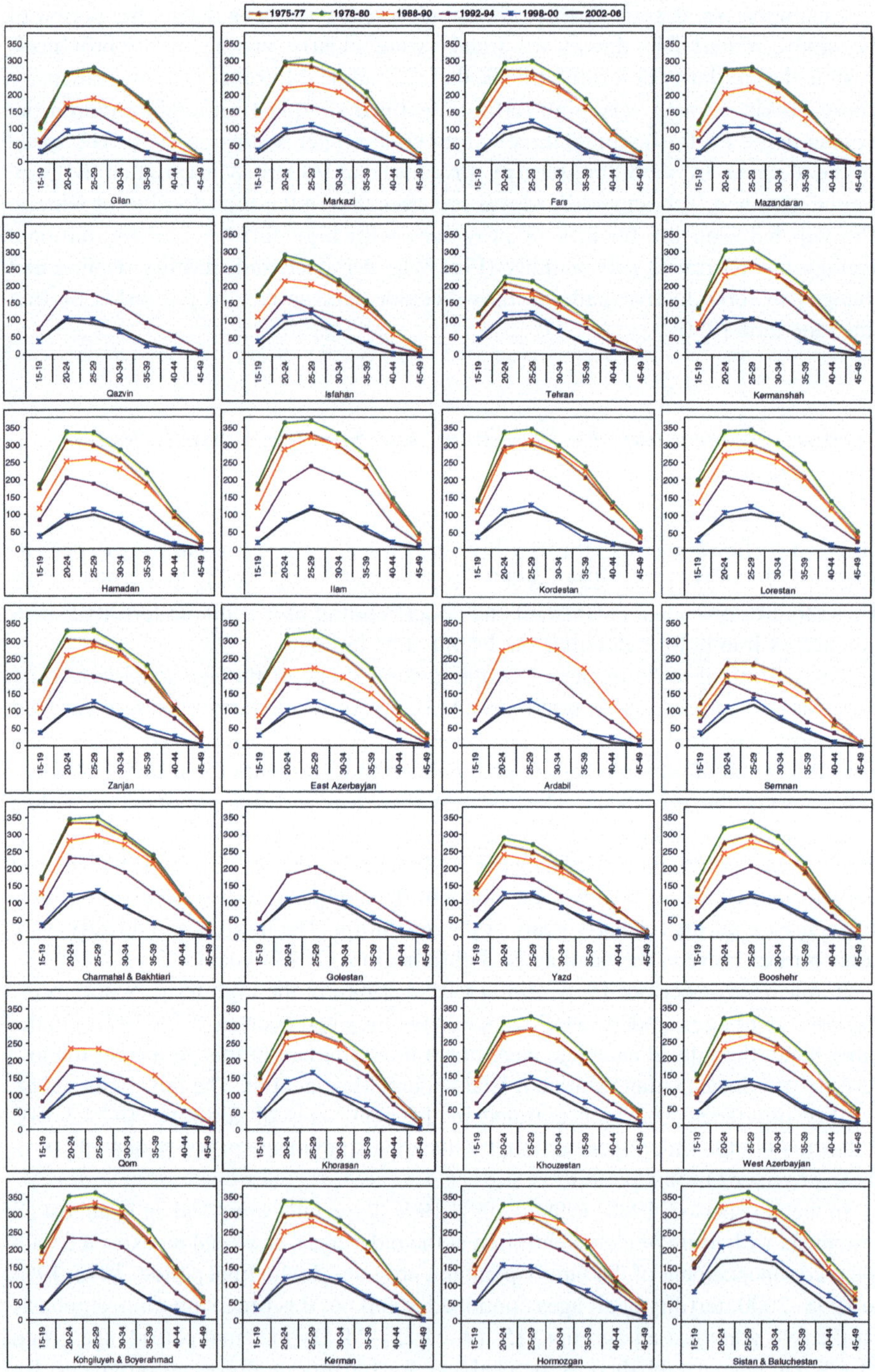

Fig. 3.6 Age specific fertility rates by province, Iran, for five 3-year periods from 1975 to 2006

Results also show that, in general, the trends of TFRs for both rural and urban areas of the provinces were identical to the national level. Although, rural areas of most provinces had very high fertility by the early 1980s, their fertility fell sharply after the re-introduction of family planning program in 1989. The decline during the 1990s in rural areas was substantial and the age patterns of fertility in both areas of the same province are more-or-less similar.

Attainment of Below-Replacement Fertility

Signs of the attainment of below-replacement fertility in Iran appeared in the first-half of the 1990s. The four developed provinces of Gilan, Semnan, Tehran and Isfahan had reached a TFR below replacement level by the period 1994–1996 (Abbasi-Shavazi 2001a). The IDHS results also revealed that, by the end of the 1990s, below-replacement fertility was no longer the exception as around 50% of provinces had had that experience. In 2006, a majority of provinces were experiencing below-replacement fertility. Gilan recorded the lowest fertility in 2006, 1.2 births per woman close to the lowest rates in the very low fertility countries of Europe and East Asia. The TFRs in Mazandaran (1.4), Isfahan, Markazi and Hamadan (1.6) were the next lowest. Lower fertility was also apparent among other provinces as, out of 30 provinces, 18 provinces had TFRs below 2.1 children per woman. Five provinces had just replacement level fertility (2.1), and only five other provinces had TFRs between 2.2 and 2.6. Only Sistan and Baluchistan (3.7) had a TFR above 3.0. By the late 1990s, the low fertility pattern was not only characteristic of highly developed provinces or urban areas but was also evident in some, more remote rural areas. Our results show that in 2006 the TFRs were below 2.1 in the urban parts of 24 provinces while only five provinces had urban TFRs between 2.1 and 2.4. TFR remained high (3.6) in only the urban areas of Sistan and Baluchistan. Similarly, in rural areas, 15 provinces had TFRs below 2.1 while 13 provinces had TFRs between 2.1 and 3.0. Only rural areas of the two provinces of Sistan and Baluchistan and Hormozgan had TFRs that were above 3.0 (Abbasi-Shavazi et al. 2008).

Summary of Fertility Trends

While differences in levels of fertility are still evident across the country, the now smaller differences reflect those that already existed in the mid 1970s. The extent and speed of the fertility decline has been a nationwide phenomenon affecting all provinces, rural and urban in much the same way. The transition has been socially inclusive, that is, all provinces, regardless of their level of socio-economic development and their distance from the capital city, followed trends and patterns broadly similar to the national average across the periods. The few provinces that still have relatively high fertility tend to have small population numbers so that the effect of their high fertility on the national average is not very substantial. There is also a geographic pattern of fertility in Iran. Provinces located on the borders of the country are those that have had very high fertility, while provinces in the central part of Iran, particularly those close to the capital, Tehran, have displayed lower fertility. This provincial level pattern extends back at least to the mid-1970s.

The consistency of these provincial differences across time suggests that their origins are cultural (ethnicity and sect of religion). It seems likely that long-standing cultural differences between regions play a role in accounting for differences in the receptivity of contraceptive use and lower fertility but it is difficult to demonstrate such influences in a conclusive or quantitative manner. The results of the Iran Fertility Transition Survey (Abbasi-Shavazi et al. 2003) are also suggestive of the potentially important role played by cultural factors in explaining differences in fertility across provinces. Other studies in Iran have confirmed the relationship between ethnicity and sect of religion and fertility (Hosseini 2008; Hosseini and Abbasi-Shavazi, 2009; Sadeghi 2004; Zanjani and Naseri 1996). Nevertheless, the ubiquitous nature of fertility change over the past three decades means that common features within Iranian society that have facilitated the rapid spread of reproductive changes across provincial boundaries need to be identified.

The provinces now emerging with very low fertility rates are those in the north-central part of Iran especially the provinces that border the Caspian Sea. As other provinces have tended to follow the patterns established in these provinces, the prospect for very low fertility across Iran is real.

References

Abbasi-Shavazi MJ (1999) Advantages and problems of the own-children method of estimating fertility using census data. J Popul (Persian) 29–30:1–21

Abbasi-Shavazi MJ (2000) National trends and social inclusion: fertility trends and differentials in the Islamic Republic of Iran. Paper presented at the IUSSP conference on family planning in the 21st century, Dhaka, 16–21 January 2000

Abbasi-Shavazi MJ (2001a) Assessment of the own-children method of estimating fertility in Iran using 1986 and 1996 censuses. Social Sci J (Persian) 16(2):105–135

Abbasi-Shavazi MJ (2001b) Below replacement fertility in Iran: progress and prospects. Paper presented at the workshop on low fertility in advanced countries: trends, theories and policies, Tokyo, 21–23 March 2001

Abbasi-Shavazi MJ (2002a) Convergence of fertility behaviours in Iran: provincial fertility levels, trends and patterns in Iran. Social Sci J (Persian) 18:201–231

Abbasi-Shavazi MJ (2002b) Recent changes and the future of fertility in Iran. Paper presented at the expert group meeting on continuing fertility transition, Population Division of the United Nations, New York, pp. 425–439

Abbasi-Shavazi MJ, Hosseini-Chavoshi M, McDonald P (2007) The path to below replacement fertility in the Islamic Republic of Iran. Asia-Pacific Popul J 22(2):91–112

Abbasi-Shavazi MJ, McDonald P (2005) National and provincial-level fertility trends in Iran: 1972–2000. Working Paper in Demography, No. 94. The Australian National University, Canberra

Abbasi-Shavazi MJ, McDonald P (2006) The fertility decline in the Islamic Republic of Iran, 1972–2000. Asian Popul Stud 2(3):217–237

Abbasi-Shavazi MJ, Hosseini-Chavoshi M, Delavar B, Aghajanian A, Mehryar A (2004b) Unintended pregnancies in the Islamic Republic of Iran: levels and correlates. Asia-Pacific Popul J 19(1):27–38

Abbasi-Shavazi MJ, McDonald P, Hosseini Chavoshi M (2003) Changes in Family, Fertility Behavior and Attitudes in Iran. Working Paper in Demography No. 88. Australian National University, Canberra

Abbasi-Shavazi MJ, Mehryar A, Jones G, McDonald P (2002) Revolution, war and modernization: population policy and fertility change in Iran. J Popul Res 19(1):25–46

Abbasi-Shavazi MJ, Sadeghi R (2006) Ethnicity and fertility: analysis of fertility behavior of ethnic groups in Iran (Persian). J Social Sci 29:29–63

Abbasi-Shavazi MJ, Hosseini-Chavoshi M, Nourollahi T (2008) Estimation and assessment of the levels and trends of fertility in Iran using the own-children method. Paper presented at the statistical center of Iran's conference on the results of the 2006 Census, Tehran, 24–25 December 2008

Agha H (1985) Study of fertility in Iran and its relation with socio-economic indicators based on the Iran fertility survey (Persian). Population Studies Center, University of Shiraz, Shiraz

Aghajanian A (1991) Population change in Iran, 1966–86: a stalled demographic transition? Popul Dev Rev 17:703–715

Aghajanian A (1995) A new direction in population policy and family planning in the Islamic Republic of Iran. Asia-Pacific Popul J 10(1):3–20

Aghajanian A, Gross AB, Lewis SM (1992) Evaluation of Iran Fertility Survey, WP 93-2. University of Washington, Center for Studies in Demography and Ecology

Aghajanian A, Mehryar AH (1999) Fertility transition in the Islamic Republic of Iran: 1967–1996. Asia-Pacific Popul J 14(1):21–42

Amani M (1996) An attempt on historical outlook of the trends of births and death rates and study of the stage of demographic transition in Iran (Persian). J Popul 13–14:71–83

Amani M (1970) Births and fertility in Iran, division of Population research (Persian). Institute for Social Studies and Research, University of Tehran, Tehran

Arnold F, Sultan M (1992) Fertility, In Pakistan demographic and health Survey, National Institute of Population Studies, Colombia, pp. 35–52

Bongaarts J, Potter RG (1983) Fertility, biology, and behavior: an analysis of the proximate determinants. Academic, New York

Cho LJ (1973) The own-children approach to fertility estimation: an elaboration. In: International population conference, Liege. International Union for the Scientific Study of Population, Liege, pp 263–279

Cho LJ, Retherford RD, Choe MK (1986) The own-children method of fertility estimation. University of Hawaii Press, Honolulu, HI

Coale AJ, Freedman R (1993) Similarities in the fertility transition in China and three other East Asian populations. In: Leete R, Alam I (eds) The revolution in Asian fertility: dimensions, causes, and implications. Clarendon Press, Oxford, pp 208–238

Eaton JW, Mayer AJ (1953) The social biology or very high fertility among the Hutterites: the demography of a unique population. Hum Biol 25(3):206–264

Fargues P (1989) The decline of Arab fertility. Population 44(1):147–175

Grabill WH, Cho LJ (1965) Methodology for the measurement of current fertility from population data on young children. Demography 2:50–73

Hakim A (2001) Fertility transition and differentials in Pakistan. In: Proceedings of the population association of Pakistan's conference on Pakistan's population: issues in the 21st century, Karachi, 24 Oct 2000, pp 611–633

Hosseini H (2008) Ethnicity and fertility: explanation of fertility behaviors among Turks and Kurds in Orumieh district. Ph.D. thesis in demography, Department of Demography, University of Tehran (Persian)

Hosseini H, Abbasi-Shavazi MJ (2009) Ideational change and its impact on fertility ideals and behaviour of Kurd and Turk women. J Women's Res [Persian]

Hosseini-Chavoshi M, McDonald P, Abbasi-Shavazi MJ (2006) The Iranian fertility decline, 1981–1999: an application of the synthetic parity progression ratio method. Population 61(5–6):701–718

Jain SK (1989) Estimation of aboriginal fertility, 1971–86: an application of the own-children method of fertility estimation. Australian Bureau of Statistics, Canberra

Kaveh-Firouz Z, Abbasi-Shavazi MJ (2004) Population policy change and its impacts on fertility trends in Iran (Persian). In: Proceeding of the 1st conference of the population association of Iran, Tehran, pp 371–396

Keshtkar M (2000) Age heaping in the 1996 Census. Population (Persian) 31–32(1):101–118

Knodel J, Chanaratrithirong A, Debavalya N (1987) Thailand's reproductive revolution: Rapid fertility decline in a third world setting. Madison: The University of Wisconsin Press

Koosheshi M (1994) Preliminary hypothesis on fertility changes in Iran [Persian]. J Popul 7:39–56

Ladier-Fouladi M (1997) The fertility transition in Iran. Popul: Engl Sel 9:191–214

Leete R, Alam I (1997) Population, socio-economic and health statistics of the Islamic republic of Iran. Unpublished Report, New York: United Nations Population Fund

Mehryar AH, Tajdini F (1998) Population and development in the Islamic Republic of Iran: a review of the main findings of the 1996 Census and other sources of data. Working Paper, Institute for Research on Planning and Development, Tehran

Mehryar AH, Gholipour R (1995a) The rise and fall of fertility rates of Iranian population after the Islamic revolution. Working Paper. Institute for Research on Planning and Development, Tehran

Mehryar AH, Gholipour R (1995b) Provincial differences in fertility in Iran, 1976–1991. Working Paper. Institute for Research on Planning and Development, Tehran

Mirzaie M (2005) Swings in fertility limitations in Iran. Critique: Crit Middle East Stud 14(1):25–33

Mirzaie M, Koosheshi M, Naseri MB (1996) Estimation and analysis of vital-demographic indicators of Iran, 1986 and 1991 (Persian). Institute of Research and Social Studies, University of Tehran, Tehran (Persian)

Nourollahi T (2000) Estimation of the levels and trends of fertility in Iran using the own-children method, 1972–1996 (Persian). MA thesis, Department of Demography, University of Tehran

Padidar-Nia, H. 1977. Population dynamics in Iran: new estimates on mortality and fertility. Ph.D. thesis, University Microfilms International, Ann Arbor, MI

Peng X (1993) Regional differentials in China's fertility transition. In: Leete R, Alam I (eds) The revolution in Asian fertility: dimensions, causes, and implications. Clarendon Press, Oxford, pp 99–127

Population Division of the Department of Economic and Social Affairs of the United Nations Secretariat (2009). World population prospects: the 2008 revision. Highlights. United Nations, New York

Rashad H (2000) Demographic transition in Arab countries: a new perspective. J Popul Res 17(1):81–101

Retherford RD, Pejaranonda C, Cho LJ, Chamratrithirong A, Arnold F (1979) Own-children estimates of fertility for Thailand based on the 1970 Census. East-West Center, Honolulu, HI

Rindfuss RR (1977) Methodological difficulties encountered in using own-children data: illustration from the United States. East-West Center, Honolulu, HI

Sadeghi R (2004) Ethnicity and fertility: explanation of fertility behaviors among ethnic groups in Iran. MA thesis in Demography, Department of Demography, University of Tehran, Tehran

Salehi-Isfahani Dj, Tandon A (2000) Fertility transition or intertemporal substitution in post-revolutionary Iran? Evidence from household data, mimeo, Department of Economics, Virginia Polytechnic Institute and State University

Saraie H (1997) Demographic transition of Iran: a preliminary report (Persian). J Social Sci 9 (Winter issue):1–18

Saraie H (1995) On the appropriateness of Whipple's index for evaluation of quality of population statistics in the Iranian population censuses. Population (Persian) 13–14:25–38

Statistical Center of Iran (1999) Results of the population growth estimation survey, first phase 1998–99. Tehran (Persian)

United Nations Fund for Population Activities (1998) Country assessment report, UNFPA, Tehran

Zanjani H (1993) A study of fertility in Iran, Centre for Urban Studies and Research, Ministry of Housing and Urban Planning, Tehran (Persian)

Zanjani H, Naseri MB (1996) Study of ethnic fertility differentials among women in Iran, Centre for Urban Studies and Research, Ministry of Housing and Urban Planning, Tehran (Persian)

Chapter 4
Fertility Dynamics Using Parity Progression Ratios*

Introduction

The cross-sectional or synthetic parity progression model provides an alternative to conventional age-based approaches to the study of fertility trends. Instead of examining births by age of mother, this method examines fertility trends according to the number of births that a women has had already (parity) in association with the time since the most recent birth (Feeney 1983; Ni-Bhrolchain 1987; Feeney and Yu 1987; Rallu and Toulemon 1994; Hinde 1998). The approach allows an interpretation of time trends in fertility in terms of the number of births individual women are having. It has also been argued that analysis by parity facilitates interpretation of fertility trends because people make their decisions about having a child on the basis of the number of children that they already have rather than simply upon how old they are.

In this chapter, synthetic cohort parity measures are examined at the national level using the 2000 Iran Demographic and Health Survey, and at the provincial level using the 2005 Iran Low Fertility Survey for four selected low fertility regions. The chapter begins with an analysis of the progression to marriage. Marriage trends are considered in more detail in Chapter 5.

The Progression to First Marriage

The legal age at first marriage was lowered soon after the Islamic revolution. In apparent response, the proportion marrying at the youngest ages increased a little between 1975 and 1980 (Fig. 4.1). As the 1980s progressed, the spread of universal high school education for girls countered this trend such that there was a sharp drop in the (synthetic cohort) proportion of girls marrying by age 18, especially between 1980 (66%) and 1986 (49%). However, at ages 20 and over, marriage rates rose between 1987 and 1990 as part of a mini marriage boom following the end of the

---

*The material presented in this chapter are drawn from Hosseini-Chavoshi (2007) and appeared as Hosseini-Chavoshi et al. (2006). The detailed methodology is set out in these references.

M.J. Abbasi-Shavazi et al., *The Fertility Transition in Iran: Revolution and Reproduction*,

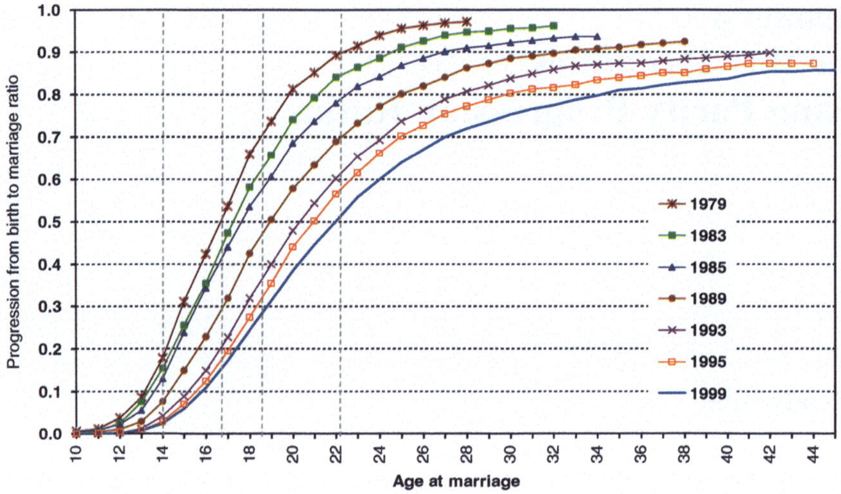

Fig. 4.1 Cumulative progression to first marriage for synthetic cohorts, Iran, 1981–1999, selected years (2000 Iran Demographic and Health Survey)

Iran–Iraq War. As discussed below, the increased rates of marriage in the last years of the 1980s served to hold annual fertility at a higher level than would otherwise have been the case during those years because births were brought forward in time.

During the 1990s, age at first marriage continued to increase gradually as more women pursued post-school education. Over the period from 1981 to 1999, the synthetic lifetime proportion ever marrying fell from 99% to 86%. It needs to be pointed out that, in a period when marriage is being delayed, this 'lifetime' measure will overstate the proportion of women that never marry. Based on preference data and observed proportions ever married for age cohorts, it can be argued that the lifetime percentage ever married for any actual cohort of Iranian women will be at least 95% for all Iranian women aged 20 and over in 1999. This means that, the effect of the timing distortion upon the synthetic proportion who ever marry was significant at the end of the 1990s. Underlining the complexity of these trends, however, it is expected that the coming to marriageable age of the very large birth cohorts of the early 1980s will lead to a further delay of marriage after 2000. This cohort will face both considerable economic problems due to competition in the labour and housing markets and considerable adjustment in the marriage market given the imbalances that will arise from huge shifts in the numbers in successive birth cohorts.

Progression to the First Birth (from Marriage)

Studies in developing countries (Westoff and Akinrinola 2001) show that around 2% of women are infertile and do not progress to their first child during their reproductive life. The results for Iran as a whole from IDHS 2000 (Fig. 4.2) show that the lifetime progression from marriage to the first birth fell across time from

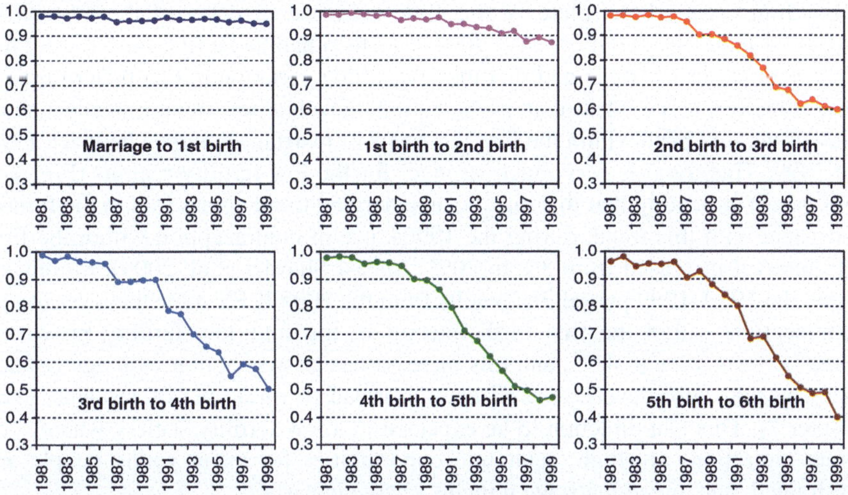

Fig. 4.2 Lifetime parity progression ratios, synthetic cohorts, Iran, 1981–1999 (2000 Iran Demographic and Health Survey)

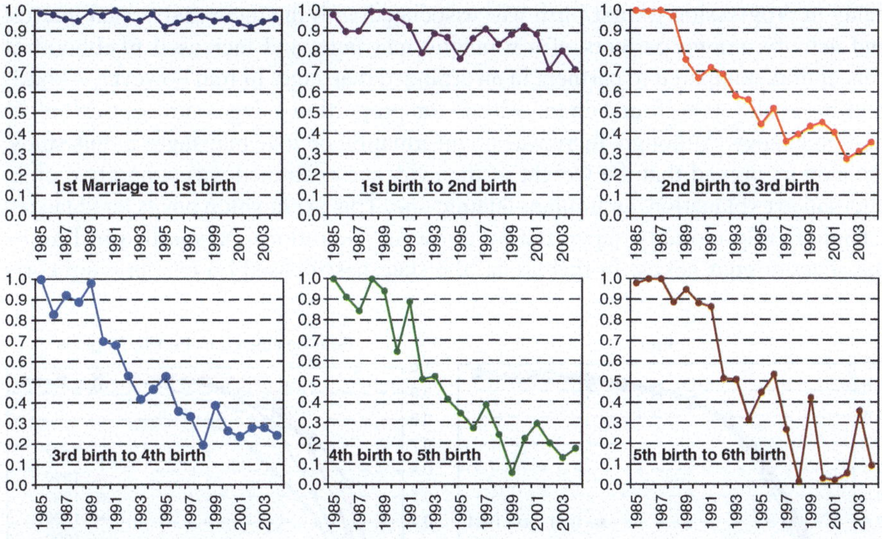

Fig. 4.3 Lifetime parity progression ratios, synthetic cohorts, four selected low fertility regions, 1981–1999 (2000 Iran Low Fertility Survey)

98% in 1981 to 95% in 1999, still at a high level at the end of the period. Hence, there was little change across time in the propensity to have a first birth. The same was true for the four low fertility provinces (Fig. 4.3). Thus, it can be concluded that fertility decline in Iran and even in the low fertility provinces has not been a consequence of married women opting to have no children.

For Iran, as a whole, there is also little evidence of delay of the first birth. Figure 4.4 indicates that more than 90% of women had had a first birth during the first 5 years after marriage and that there was little variation in this pattern across time. However, it is evident that, at the national level, a new trend towards a short delay of the first birth within the first few years of marriage emerged between 1996 and 1999. This trend is very much stronger for the low fertility regions (Fig. 4.4, right panel) indicating that this may be an emerging trend across Iran in the future. Consistent with this trend, during the 1990s, use of contraception within the first birth interval increased from 3% to 20% (Abbasi-Shavazi et al. 2009). Moreover, during the 1980–1999 period, the results from the 2005 ILFS show that ever use of contraception within the first birth interval in the four low fertility provinces increased from 14% to 41%, and this increase has an association with age at marriage and education levels, as well as with urban or rural area of residence (see Chapter 7). This is a direction to be expected in a low fertility society where economic aspirations are high, economic opportunities for many young people are constrained, and age at marriage remains relatively early.

Rindfuss and Morgan (1983) found that in several Asian countries romantic marriage has increased and arranged marriage has decreased, and that couples married through romantic marriage were less likely to delay their first child as compared with those married through an arranged marriage. They argued that less delay in progression to first birth was associated with the increased sexual interest and activity among partners of a romantic marriage, and increased likelihood of conception, compared to partners in an arranged marriage. In Iran however, Abbasi-Shavazi et al. (2009) found an increase in the proportion using contraception before first pregnancy. Although, there was no information on love marriages in this study, the authors argued that the weight of the evidence examined was supportive of an alternative explanation, an Iranian–Islamic one. This explanation posits an idealized Islamic family morality supported by powerful institutions, personified in Iran by the state/religion nexus. In this arena, the state has focused on encouraging early

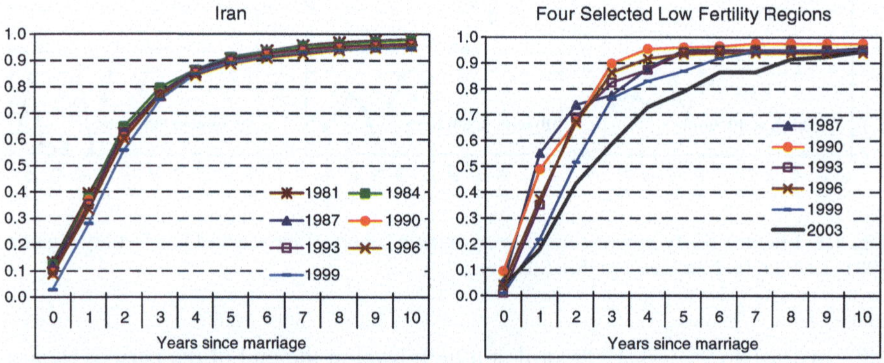

Fig. 4.4 Cumulative parity progression, synthetic cohorts, marriage to first birth, Iran and four low fertility provinces, 1981–2003, selected years (2000 Iran Demographic and Health Survey; 2005 Iran Low Fertility Survey)

marriage and provides resources for doing so. As a result individuals turn to birth control early in marriage to conform to early marriage expectations while postponing parenthood. This explanation sees the new behaviour as conservative, maintaining earlier marriage than would be expected without state/religious influence.

Further, the increase in contraceptive use prior to the first child in recent years is compatible with the program implemented by the Ministry of Health by which newly married couples are required to attend marriage counselling sessions prior to first marriage. The program provides them with comprehensive knowledge and information about contraception and health and social aspects of motherhood and fatherhood. This program aims to educate couples about delaying their first child.

In general, despite this emerging delay of the first birth, it can be concluded that delaying the first child did not contribute significantly to fertility decline in Iran up to the year, 2000.

Progression to the Second Birth

Lifetime progression to the second birth for Iranian women (Fig. 4.2) was very high in the early years of the revolution (99%), fell slowly to 1990 (97%) and then more sharply in the 1990s to 87% in 1999. Similar results are observed for the low fertility provinces in Fig. 4.3. Lifetime progression to the second birth for women in the four selected provinces was very high during the period 1985–1989 (around 99%), fell slowly, though with some fluctuations, to around 92% in 1990, and then with some yearly fluctuation fell to around 88 by 1999. However, after 1999, in the low fertility provinces, the lifetime percentage progressing to a second birth fell sharply to around 70% by the period 2002–2004. It is not suggested that 30% of women in these provinces will not progress from the first to the second birth. Instead, this trend reflects a substantial increase in the interval between the first and the second birth.

In what is probably one of the most significant findings of this chapter, Fig. 4.5 shows the onset of a very substantial delay of the second birth. For example, the proportion of Iranian women having their second birth within 3.5 years of their first birth fell from 81% in 1981 to 72% in 1990 and then to 34% in 1999. The difference between the 1981 and 1999 figures in the third year after the first birth (47% points) is much wider than the corresponding difference in the 10th year after the first birth (12% points). This means that what is being observed here is wider spacing of the interval between the – first and second births, rather than a 'stopping at one' pattern. Thus, for any real cohort, the percentages of women who stop at one may not be as high as 13% for Iran as a whole or 30% for the low fertility provinces. On the other hand, the results of the 2002 Iran Fertility Transition Survey on preferences of women confirm an emerging trend in some parts of the country (Abbasi-Shavazi et al. 2003; 2004). Note that in the province of Gilan the tendency to have one child only has been high even for those who

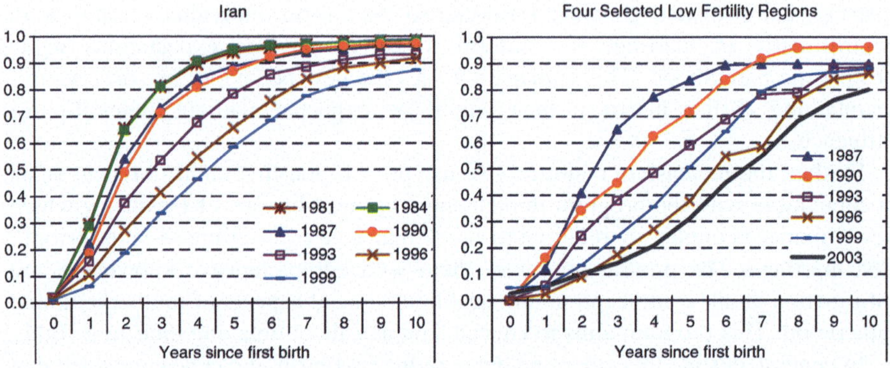

Fig. 4.5 Cumulative parity progression, synthetic cohorts, first birth to the second birth, Iran and four low fertility provinces, 1981–2003, selected years (2000 Iran Demographic and Health Survey; 2005 Iran Low Fertility Survey)

married before the 1980s. The level has increased from around 18% to around 22.5% for recent cohorts (see Chapter 8).

Progression to the second birth is very slow in the low fertility provinces. In 2003, only 30% progressed to the second birth within 5 years after the first birth and the 50% mark was reached after 7 years. These are extraordinarily long birth intervals. This can be explained by the fact that most Iranian women are still quite young when they have their first birth and the family economy not very advanced. The Iranian solution to this problem is to delay the second birth to an extent hardly observed in any other country. The continued lengthening of the interval to the second birth would have had the effect of forcing down the annual fertility rate as births were postponed to a future time (a timing or tempo effect). The longer birth intervals do not cost Iranian families as much as they would in some other countries (Groat et al. 1976; Jones 1984; Hoem 1993; Evans 1996; Anderson 2000), because of the low labour force participation rate for women in Iran (Mehryar and Farjadi 2000; Mahmoudian 2006).

The timing of the widening of the second birth interval corresponds closely with the reintroduction of the nationwide family planning program in Iran. Prior to 1990, there is little evidence of a change in the interval between the first and the second birth suggesting that this was not an explanation of the movements in fertility from the mid 1970s to the late 1980s.

Progression to the Third Birth

It is with progression to the third birth that we begin to observe the substantial changes in the quantum of fertility. In the early 1980s, the synthetic lifetime measure shows that 96–97% of women in Iran who had had a second child continued to the third. By 1999, this had fallen to 60% (Fig. 4.2). The results of the Iran Low Fertility Survey in Fig. 4.3 also show that during 1985–1987 almost all women in the four provinces who had a second child continued to have the third child but this figure had declined to around 56% in 1984, before it fell to around 30% during 2002–2004.

The trend over the period closely mirrored the trend in the total fertility rate (see Chapter 3) – high in the early 1980s, a slow decline to 1990 and more rapid decline thereafter. It is very evident that 'stopping at two' is the central story of fertility decline in Iran. It is also evident that this new pattern had commenced prior to the reestablishment of the family planning program. Thus, the family planning program can be considered to have facilitated and accelerated a pattern of behaviour that had become established in parts of the society in the mid 1980s. Abbasi-Shavazi et al. (2003) based on analysis of the 2002 Iran Fertility Transition Survey proposed that the economic aspirations of the population were raised by the revolution but the failure of household economic outcomes to meet expectations had become clearly evident by the mid 1980s.

In addition, it was evident to parents by the mid 1980s that their children would have better opportunities for education and social advancement in the new society if the parents were able to support their children through education. Stopping at two must have been seen by parents as a strategy to improve their own economic outcomes and the educational opportunities of their children (Abbasi-Shavazi et al. 2004). The interesting question becomes what means of fertility control did women use to stop at two before the reestablishment of the family planning program? This will be addressed in Chapter 7.

The annualised cumulative progressions (Fig. 4.6) indicate another very interesting trend not evident from age-based analyses. The emergence of 'stopping at two' seems to have been preceded by a long-term trend towards wider spacing of the second and third births, a trend that continued through the early 1980s when fertility rates

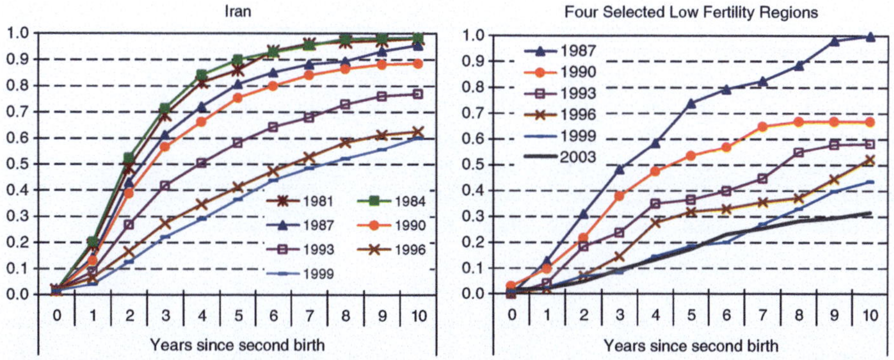

Fig. 4.6 Cumulative parity progression, synthetic cohorts, second birth to the third birth, Iran and four low fertility provinces, 1981–2003, selected years (2000 Iran Demographic and Health Survey; 2005 Iran Low Fertility Survey)

were at their highest. For example, based on the 1975–1979 cross-sections, 54% of women had moved from their second to their third birth by the end of the second year; for the 1980–1984 cross-sections, at the height of the high fertility, 49% had done so. This percentage then declines further in subsequent years. This may mean either that couples were already attempting unsuccessfully to stop at two or that they were indeed attempting to widen the interval between the second and third birth.

Movement to the third birth has been slower among women in low fertility regions for all birth cohorts as shown in the right panel of Fig. 4.6. For the 1987 cross-sections, before the revival of the family planning program, 30% had moved from their second to their third birth by the end of the second year, but less than 8% had done so since 1999. More importantly, the life time progression to the third birth in the low fertility provinces fell from near 100% in 1987 to 30% by 2003.

Progression to the Fourth and Higher Order Births

The phenomenon of 'stopping at two' from 1986 onwards extends to higher parities in the sense that, if a woman already had more than two children, there was an increased tendency across time to stop at whatever her parity was (Figs. 4.2 and 4.3 and Table 4.1). Between 1986 and 1990, largely before the impact of the family planning program, the tendency to stop increased as parity increased for Iranian women. This pattern was accentuated between 1990 and 1999 with the family planning program in operation.

Table 4.1 Life time parity progression ratios, synthetic parity cohorts, ever married women, Iran and four selected low fertility provinces, 1981–2003

Parity progression	Lifetime percentage progressing										
	1981	1983	1986	1988	1990	1992	1995	1997	1999	2001	2003
Iran (national level)[a]											
Marriage to 1st	98.0	97.2	97.8	96.1	96.3	96.6	96.6	96.2	94.9		
1st to 2nd	98.6	99.3	98.7	97.0	97.4	94.8	90.9	87.6	87.4		
2nd to 3rd	98.2	97.5	97.8	90.5	88.7	82.0	68.1	64.2	60.3		
3rd to 4th	98.9	98.4	95.8	89.3	89.9	77.4	63.6	59.3	50.3		
4th to 5th	97.9	97.9	96.0	90.1	86.2	71.2	56.7	49.7	47.2		
5th to 6th	96.4	94.6	96.2	92.8	84.1	68.4	54.9	48.7	40.1		
Combined four selected low fertility provinces [b]											
Marriage to 1st			98.1	94.9	97.7	95.9	92.1	96.5	94.8	93.8	94.5
1st to 2nd			89.7	99.5	96.5	79.3	76.4	90.7	88.1	88.3	80.1
2nd to 3rd			99.5	97.3	67.1	68.9	44.7	36.3	43.6	40.7	31.6
3rd to 4th			83.0	88.8	69.8	53.0	52.6	33.2	38.6	23.6	27.9

[a] 2000 Iran Demographic and Health Survey.
[b] 2005 Iran Low Fertility Survey.

Figures 4.7 and 4.8 confirm the strong cross-sectional pattern of stopping at whatever parity a woman had at the time. The largest shift occurs in the early years of the family planning program (between 1990 and 1993) suggesting that there was a considerable unmet need for contraception that was satisfied with enthusiasm as soon as this option was provided. The cumulated proportion of women having a fourth birth during 1985–1988 was between 90% and 99% but this figure fell to less than 50% for the whole country by 1999.

Lifetime progression to the fourth birth in the late 1980s in the low fertility regions was almost the same as observed at the national level, and around 90% of women progressed to their fourth birth. However, after 1990, lifetime progression to the fourth birth is much lower among women in the low fertility provinces than at the national level being, for example, 70% at the national level compared with 40% in

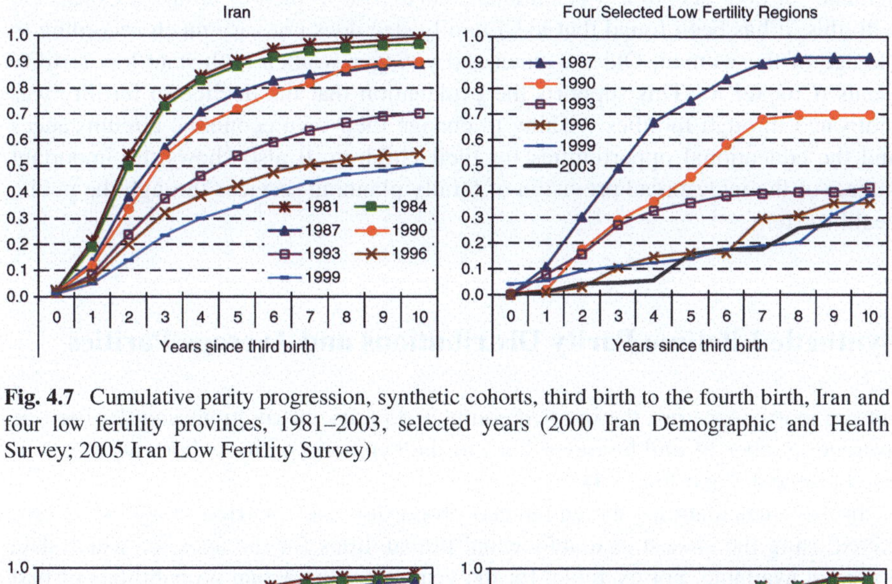

Fig. 4.7 Cumulative parity progression, synthetic cohorts, third birth to the fourth birth, Iran and four low fertility provinces, 1981–2003, selected years (2000 Iran Demographic and Health Survey; 2005 Iran Low Fertility Survey)

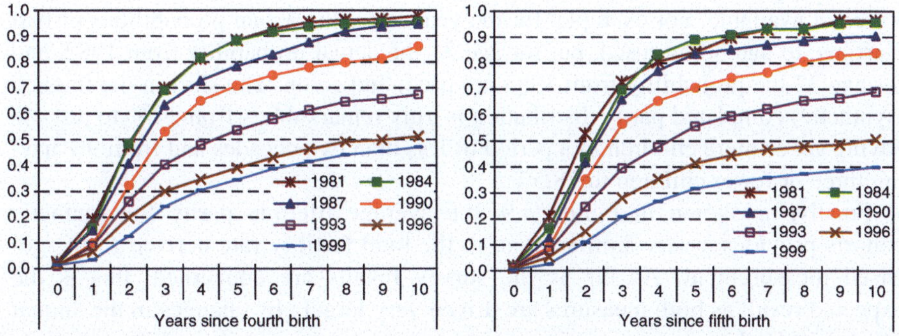

Fig. 4.8 Cumulative parity progression, synthetic cohorts, fourth to the fifth birth and fifth to the sixth birth, Iran, 1981–1999, selected years (2000 Iran Demographic and Health Survey)

the low fertility regions for the 1993 birth cohort. By 2003, the cumulated progression to the fourth birth had fallen to as low as 20% in the low fertility regions.

By 2003, in the low fertility regions, the rates of progression to the third and fourth births were as low as the equivalent progressions in countries of Europe that have very low fertility rates (Italy, Spain, Austria) and well below those European countries such as France and Sweden that have moderately low fertility. That what was happening was stopping behaviour rather than spacing behaviour is indicated by the fact that the fall in lifetime parity progression ratios is very similar to the fall by the third year after the previous birth. Thus, the lifetime parity progression ratios for all births beyond the second birth are unlikely to be affected much by delaying of these births.

From a theoretical perspective, it is evident that stopping behaviour was very strongly cross-sectional. Stopping was not a phenomenon that emerged gradually with successive cohorts, for example, through increasing levels of education. The demand for contraception was simultaneous across women of all ages. Consistent with this, it has been found that ideal family size does not vary much according to the age of the woman. Older women and younger women both state low fertility ideals (Chapter 8). This supports the explanation that the decline in fertility was motivated through families wishing to change their own economic circumstances and the educational opportunities for their children. It also shows the important impact of the widespread provision of family planning services through the public health system.

Synthetic Lifetime Parity Distributions and Average Parities

As summary measures, the implied completed parity distributions and the lifetime average number of children ever born to the synthetic parity cohorts were calculated (Table 4.2 and Fig. 4.9).

In these calculations, the cumulated proportion ever married to age 49 is projected using the closest available actual probabilities for the ages for which data were not available. For example, for the year 1981, the actual probabilities of first marriage to age 30 are used, but for age 31 the actual probability from 1982, and for age 32 the probability from 1983 are used, and so on. The shift in the implied (synthetic) completed parity distribution is truly remarkable – from 86% to just 4% having six or more children in a period of less than two decades and from 9% having three or fewer children to 78.5%.

Finally, as shown in Figure 4.9, the average lifetime parity for synthetic cohorts provides a very similar trend to the total fertility rate derived from age-based measurement. As far as the survey results are concerned, this is the expected result as both measures are driven very largely by changes in the annual number of births.

Table 4.2 Implied completed parity distribution and life time average parity, Synthetic parity cohorts, Iran and four selected low fertility provinces, 1981–2003

	Lifetime percentage progressing										
Parity progression	1981	1983	1986	1988	1990	1992	1995	1997	1999	2001	2003
Iran (National level)[a]											
0 (Non-marriage)	2.9	3.8	6.8	8.1	5.4	10.1	12.6	14.3	14.2		
0 (Within marriage)	2.0	2.7	2.0	3.6	3.5	3.1	3.0	3.3	4.4		
1	1.4	0.7	1.2	2.6	2.4	4.5	7.7	10.2	10.3		
2	1.7	2.3	2.0	8.1	10.0	14.8	24.5	25.8	28.3		
3	1.0	1.5	3.7	8.3	7.9	15.3	19.1	18.9	21.3		
4	1.9	1.9	3.4	6.9	9.7	15.0	14.4	13.8	11.4		
5	3.2	4.7	3.0	4.5	9.7	11.7	8.5	7.0	6.1		
6+	86.0	82.4	77.9	57.8	51.3	25.4	10.3	6.7	4.1		
Total	100.0	100.0	100.0	100.0	100.0	100.0	100.0	100.0	100.0		
Average parity	6.9	6.7	6.4	5.4	5.3	3.9	2.9	2.6	2.4		
Four selected low fertility provinces [b]											
0 (Non-marriage)			13.2	12.8	2.0	11.7	6.2	10.1	8.4	3.7	18.1
0 (Within marriage)			1.6	4.4	2.2	3.6	7.4	3.1	4.7	5.9	4.5
1			8.7	0.4	3.4	17.5	20.4	8.0	10.3	10.6	15.4
2			0.4	2.3	30.4	20.9	36.5	50.1	43.2	47.3	42.4
3			12.9	8.9	18.7	21.8	14.0	19.1	20.5	24.8	14.1
4			5.5	0.0	15.3	12.0	10.2	5.8	12.2	5.4	4.8
5			0.0	8.0	3.3	6.1	3.0	2.7	0.4	2.2	0.5
6+			57.7	63.1	24.7	6.5	2.4	1.0	0.3	0.1	0.3
Total			100.0	100.0	100.0	100.0	100.0	100.0	100.0	100.0	100.0
Average parity			4.9	5.3	3.8	2.5	2.1	2.1	2.1	2.1	1.7

[a] The 2000 Iran Demographic and Health Survey.
[b] The 2005 Iran Low Fertility Survey.

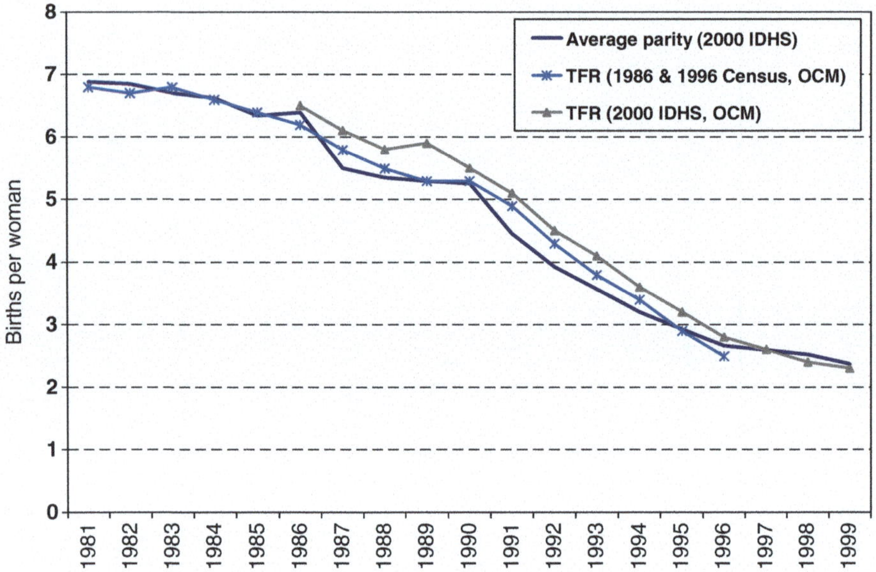

Fig. 4.9 Average lifetime parity for synthetic cohorts (Abbasi-Shavazi and McDonald 2005 [Own Children Method applied to the Iran 1986 and 1996 Censuses and the IDHS]) compared with the total fertility rate (2000 Iran Demographic and Health Survey), Iran, 1981–1999

Decomposition of Fertility

Figure 4.10 shows a decomposition of the change in the annual lifetime fertility between 1981 and 1999 into changes in the progression to marriage and the progression to each successive birth. The top line, labelled 'Woman's birth to marriage' shows the change in period lifetime fertility that would have occurred if only the probabilities of progression to marriage had changed with no change from 1981 in any of the other progressions. The second line labelled 'Marriage to first birth' then adds the additional effect of changes in the progression from marriage to first birth. Successively, other progressions are added with the final line, when progression from the fifth to the sixth birth is added, showing the actual trend in annual lifetime fertility.

The figure shows that the change in the timing of marriage on its own would have reduced the annual lifetime fertility from around 7 births to 6 births over the whole period. Changes in progression from marriage to the first birth reduce the total fertility only slightly to 5.8, and changes in progression to the second birth reduce fertility a further 0.5 births per woman to 5.3. The progressions from birth to marriage, to first birth and to second birth are the changes where timing effects will be playing a part as described earlier. Nevertheless, these trends are unlikely to turn upwards in the foreseeable future, that is, the timing effects are not likely to be short-term. Further back in time, however, the trends for these progressions display a very interesting short-term timing effect. In the final years of the 1980s, the years

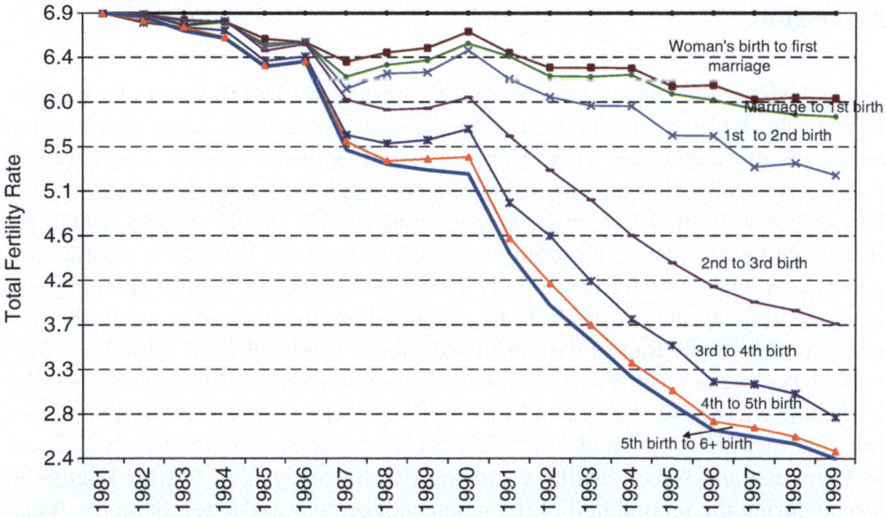

Fig. 4.10 Decomposition of the 1981–2004 declines in fertility in Iran across the progression to marriage and each successive birth (2000 Iran Demographic and Health Survey)

immediately following the end of the Iran–Iraq War, the annual progression to marriage had the effect of increasing fertility (by about 0.2 births per woman) and there was also a small upward impact from the progression from the first to the second child. These timing effects produced a kink (a flattening) in the decline of synthetic lifetime fertility between 1987 and 1990. This accentuated the apparent fall in fertility from 1990 onwards. This observation could not have been made using conventional age-based measures of fertility and shows the explanatory power of the parity progression model.

As would be expected, by far the largest impact on annual lifetime fertility is caused by the fall in progression from the second to the third birth. This commences effectively from 1988 and becomes increasingly larger with time. It accounts for a fall of around 1.6 births per woman in total. The fall in progression from the 3rd to the 4th birth is evident as early as 1984 as the first real sign of the impending fertility decline. Its effect gradually increases to 1987, levels off between 1987 and 1990 but then becomes increasingly more significant from 1990 onwards. Similar conclusions apply, at a lower level of significance, for the progression from the 4th to the 5th birth. The falls in these three progressions, from the second to the fifth birth, are most unlikely to be temporary and therefore reflect an irreversible fall in the quantum of fertility. They indicate the stopping behaviour that is central to the fall in Iran's fertility rate.

While, cessation of childbearing at parities two and above clearly has played the major role in the decline of Iranian fertility from 1986 to 2000, the emergence of very low fertility in the low fertility provinces seems to have been driven in large measure by substantial increases in the intervals between marriage and first birth and between the first birth and the second birth.

Discussion

The analysis in this chapter has shown that fertility in Iran fell so rapidly because women who had two or more children decided at much the same time to stop having any more children. There were some early signs of a desire to stop at two in the early 1980s that appear to have been largely unsuccessful but there was more success from 1986 onwards and considerably more success when the nationwide family planning programme was put in place. Fertility at parities two and over fell substantially in the early 1990s. Subsequently, family planning was also used to delay the second birth to a point where the interval between the first and second birth in Iran is extraordinarily long. Caldwell et al. (1992, p. 219) found that African fertility decline also occurred at all ages, although the speed of the decline was not as sharp as in Iran's fertility decline. This is a different picture from that identified by Knodel (1977, p. 232) as characterizing the early years of the European and Asian fertility transitions. In his analysis of fertility decline in Europe during the second half of the nineteenth century and a decade in the Asian fertility transition (mostly after 1955), he found that declines were usually nonexistent below age 25, small but increasing with age thereafter, and large only after age 40.

Finally, in recent years, especially in the low fertility provinces, there is evidence of a delay of the first birth within marriage. Delays of the first and second births would have had the effect of lowering annual even more than would have been the case if only a 'stopping at two' phenomenon was in place. The combination of the delay of first and second births and the avoidance of births beyond the second produced the spectacular decline in Iranian fertility.

The analysis indicates that the motivation to limit births was evident before the recommencement of the family planning programme in 1990 but that it was the family planning programme that enabled vast numbers of Iranians to implement their motivation to limit the number of their children. There are strong pointers from this analysis that economic motivations were paramount, that economic aspirations exceeded the capacity of families to meet their economic goals and that families considered that limiting the number of their children would assist them in meeting their goals for themselves and for their children.

References

Abbasi-Shavazi MJ, McDonald P, Hosseini-Chavoshi M (2003) Changes in family, fertility behavior and attitudes in Iran. Working paper in Demography no. 88. The Australian National University, Canberra

Abbasi-Shavazi MJ, Hosseini-Chavoshi M, McDonald PF, Delavar B (2004) Fertility transition in Iran: evidence from four selected provinces (Persian). Ministry of Health and Medical Education, Tehran

Abbasi-Shavazi MJ, McDonald PF (2005) National and provincial fertility trends in Iran, 1972–2000. Working Paper in Demography No. 94. The Australian National University, Canberra

Abbasi-Shavazi MJ, Morgan P, Hosseini-Chavoshi M, McDonald P (2009) The first birth interval in Iran: birth control use before first pregnancy. J Marriage Fam [forthcoming]

Anderson G (2000) The impact of labour-force participation on childbearing behaviour: pro-cyclical fertility in Sweden during the 1980s and the 1990s. Eur J Popul 16:293–333

Caldwell JC, Orubuloye IO, Caldwell P (1992) Fertility decline in Africa: a new type of transition? Popul Dev Rev 18(2):211–242

Evans MDR (1996) Women's labour force participation in Australia: recent research findings. J Popul Res 13(1):67–92

Feeney G (1983) Population dynamics based on birth intervals and parity progression. Popul Stud 37(1):75–89

Feeney G, Yu J (1987) Period parity measures of fertility in China. Popul Stud 41(1):77–102

Groat HT, Workman RL, Neal AG (1976) Labor force participation and family formation: a study of working mothers. Demography 13(1):115–125

Hinde A (1998) Demographic methods. Oxford University Press, New York

Hoem JM (1993) Public policy as the fuel of fertility: effects of a policy reform on the pace of childbearing in Sweden in the 1980s. Acta Sociol 36(1):19–31

Hosseini-Chavoshi M, McDonald P, Abbasi-Shavazi MJ (2006) The Iranian fertility decline, 1981–1999: an application of the synthetic parity progression ratio method. Population 61(5–6):701–718

Hosseini-Chavoshi M (2007) Fertility regulation in Iran: an analysis of trends, levels and correlates. Ph.D. thesis in Demography, Australian Demographic and Social Research Institute, The Australian National University, Canberra

Jones GW (1984) Women in the urban and industrial workforce: East and Southeast Asia. Australian National University Press, Canberra

Knodel J (1977) Family limitation and fertility transition: evidence from the age patterns of fertility in Europe and Asia. Popul Stud 31(2):219–249

Mahmoudian H (2006) Socio-demographic factors affecting women's labour force participation in Iran. Critique: Crit Middle Eastern Stud 15(3):233–248

Mehryar A, Farjadi G (2000) Labour force participation of women in Iran. Institute for Research on Planning and Development, Tehran

Ni-Bhrolchain M (1987) Period parity progression ratios and birth intervals in England and Wales, 1941–1971: a synthetic life table analysis. Popul Stud 41(1):103–125

Rallu J, Toulemon L (1994) Period fertility measures: the construction of different indices and their application to France, 1946–89. Population 6:59–93

Rindfuss RR, Morgan SP (1983) Marriage, sex, and the first birth interval: the quiet revolution in Asia. Popul Dev Rev 9:259–278

Westoff CF, Akinrinola B (2001) The contraception-fertility link in Sub-Saharan Africa and in other developing countries. ORC Macro, Calverton, MD

Chapter 5
Effects of Marital Fertility and Nuptiality on Fertility Transition in Iran, 1976–2006*

Introduction

In any study of fertility, marital status is important to the extent that it affects three stages of reproduction: intercourse, conception and parturition (VandenHeuvel and McDonald 1994, p. 69). It is generally assumed that early marriage is associated with a high proportion eventually marrying. Rising mean ages at marriage and rising percentages single are, on the other hand, associated with declines in annual measures of fertility. Later marriage reduces the total duration of fecund exposure to sexual activity, and shifts it to the older ages of lower fecundity (Smith 1983, pp. 476–80). Generally, there is an inverse relationship between the number of children ever born and age at marriage at the level of the individual couple (Knodel 1983, p. 78).

The rapid falls in fertility in East Asia (Japan, South Korea, China, Hong Kong SAR and Taiwan) and in some countries of Southeast Asia (Thailand, Singapore) were very much associated with rising age at first marriage. In the first decades of fertility decline in these countries, falls in the proportions married accounted for well over 50% of the overall fall in fertility. Ages at first marriage for women in all of these countries have risen to quite high levels with only small proportions marrying under the age of 25. In contrast, the fertility decline in Indonesia (McNicoll and Singarimbun 1981) was due primarily to falls in marital fertility with only relatively modest increases in age at first marriage. Thus, the question arises to what extent the observed fertility decline in Iran has been associated with rise in age at marriage or to lower marital fertility due to the use of contraceptives. This is the main focus of this chapter.

Using the own-children fertility estimates based on the 1986, 1996, and 2006 Censuses, the change in fertility in Iran from 1976 to 2006 is decomposed into the two main components of nuptiality and marital fertility. The proportions of women in each age group who were married are obtained from published data from the 1976, 1986, 1996 and 2006 Censuses. The analysis is based on the decomposition method of Kitagawa (1955) as adapted by Retherford and Ogawa (1978).

---

* An earlier version of the this paper was published as ANU Demography Working Paper (Abbasi-Shavazi 2000).

The 30-year change (1976–2006) in fertility for Iran and each province is decomposed into a component due to changing age-specific proportions married (nuptiality) and a component due to changing age-specific marital fertility rates. Each of these two components is further broken down by age. For the sake of convenience, the results of decomposition by age are presented only for the whole country by rural and urban areas. This chapter presents the contributions of nuptiality and marital fertility to overall fertility change during the three periods 1976–1986, 1986–1996, and 1996–2006. As discussed in Chapter 2, in these periods, there were virtually two different population policies in Iran. The first period (1976–1986) was mainly affected by pronatalist policies implemented after the 1979 Islamic Revolution whereas the second and third periods were a period of antinatalist policies introduced and executed by the government.

The results of the decomposition analysis show that during the first two periods, 1976–1986 and 1986–1996, around 85% of the change in fertility was due to falling marital fertility, that is, to control of fertility within marriage. Around 15% of the change was attributable to changes in nuptiality, specifically a reduction in the proportion of women married at younger ages. As expected, however, during the period 1996–2006, the proportion of change due to nuptiality increased to 35% and marital fertility contributed 65% to the decline of fertility.

Changes in Age at First Marriage

The extent of change in marriage is greater during the two periods 1986–1996 and 1996–2006 than in the earlier decade, 1976–1986. Table 5.1 shows the female singulate mean age at marriage (SMAM) and age-specific proportions married for the years, 1976, 1986, 1996 and 2006 for Iran. As can be seen from the table, the SMAM for Iran increased slightly from 19.7 years in 1976 to 19.8 years in 1986. This was followed by a sharper increase to 22.4 years in 1996 and 23.3 in 2006. Interestingly, the Government of Iran has consistently encouraged early marriage since 1979. During the decade after the 1979 Islamic Revolution, young couples were offered a range of incentives to marry early. The legal minimum age at marriage for girls and boys was reduced from 15 and 18 to 13 and 15 years, respectively (Azimi 1981).[1] Despite the vigorous campaign in support of early marriage, age at first marriage increased only slightly during this period. From 1976 to 1986, the proportion of women married declined moderately in all age groups except age group 20–24 for which there was a small rise. However, there was a sharp decline in proportions married in all younger age groups from 1986 to 1996 and 2006. The declines at ages 15–19 and 20–24 during 1986–1996 were substantial (Bahramitash and Kazemipour 2006). However, the decrease in proportion married at ages 20–24 and 25–29 during the last decade, 1996–2006 is also substantial.

[1] Marriage for girls aged 9 to 12 was subject to their physical development, medical approval, and legal permission from the court.

Table 5.1 Female singulate mean age at marriage (SMAM) and age specific percentages married, 1976–2006, Iran

		Percentage married in age group		
Year	SMAM	15–19	20–24	25–29
1976	19.7	34.3	78.6	93.2
1986	19.8	33.5	79.6	90.6
1996	22.4	18.6	60.7	85.2
2006	23.3	16.9	50.3	75.9

Table 5.2 Mean age at first marriage for males and females in 1980, 1990 and 2000 (calculated from the 2000 Iran Demographic and Health Survey)

	Males		Females	
Year	Rural	Urban	Rural	Urban
1980	22.3	23.2	17.0	17.8
1990	22.4	24.9	19.6	19.5
2000	24.0	25.8	19.7	20.8

Using another measure, the mean age at marriage for females also increased from 1970 to 2000 from 14.4 years (in both rural and urban areas) in 1970 to 19.7 and 20.8 in 2000 for rural and urban areas, respectively (Table 5.2). This trend is consistent with the rise of higher education among females during this period, on the one hand, and the rise in the gap between economic aspiration and reality which was discussed earlier, on the other hand. Aghajanian (1998) noted that, in terms of social norms, the proper time for a woman to marry has moved to after she has finished her high school education. This was confirmed by the results of the IFTS that showed that the majority of women in the four selected provinces preferred that their daughters continue their education rather than marrying early (Chapter 8).

Table 5.2 also compares the changes in age at marriage for men and women. The age difference between husbands and wives fell from 1980 to 2000. In rural areas for example, the difference in the mean marriage ages of men and women was 5.3 years in 1980 but 4.3 years in 2000. The lowering of the age difference between husbands and wives is an aspect of the improved autonomy of women (see Chapter 9).

Despite the increase in mean age at marriage, universal marriage is one of the major characteristics of the Iranian marriage pattern. Marriage is strongly supported by both religion and tradition in Iranian society. To get married is not only a matter of personal interest but also a duty of the young to their families and to society. As a result, the majority of women get married before age 30 and almost all women get married by their early 40s. The percentage of women ever-married at ages 35–39 declined slightly from around 98 in 1976 to around 97 in 1996, and by their late 40s, 99% of women had been married. There is a small trend to less than universal marriage recently. In 2006, around 94% of women were married at ages 35–39, and 97.8% were married by their late 40s. Although the proportion of never-married women is slightly higher for urban women, the rural–urban difference is negligible.

Table 5.3 Changes in literacy rates of the Iranian population aged 6 years and above, 1956–2006 (%) (for figures 1956–1996, Mehryar and Tajdini (1998) and for 2006, Statistical Center of Iran (2007))

	Males			Females		
Year	Total	Urban	Rural	Total	Urban	Rural
1956	22.2	45.2	10.8	14.9	20.6	1.0
1966	40.1	61.5	25.4	17.9	38.3	4.3
1976	58.8	74.4	43.6	35.6	55.7	17.4
1986	71.0	80.5	60.1	51.0	65.2	36.0
1996	84.7	89.6	76.7	74.2	81.7	62.4
2006	88.7	92.2	76.7	80.3	85.5	69.0

The change in marriage patterns in the provinces of Iran was similar to the national level, a slower pace during 1976–1986, and a major change during 1986–1996 followed by another change during 1996–2006. In general, SMAM increased by more than 2 years in most provinces. However, provincial differences in mean age at marriage were still very evident in 1996: the highest SMAM was recorded for Gilan (23.4 years), while the lowest figure related to Sistan and Baluchistan (20.4 years).

The change in marriage pattern is consistent with other socio-economic changes in the Islamic Republic of Iran over the last two decades. As discussed in Chapter 2, the increased educational attainment of Iranian women during the last two decades is very notable. Female literacy for the age group 6 years and above increased from 15% in 1956 to 35% in 1976, to 74% in 1996, and to 80% in 2006 (Table 5.3). The school enrolment rate of the female population has also increased in this period and the parents of young women prefer them to finish high school at least before marrying. Many more young women than young men are continuing to post-school education as well. Rapid urbanisation has meant that young couples in urban areas face high housing costs and economic pressure has also been a major factor in the postponement of marriage. As discussed in Chapter 2, Iran experienced economic hardship after the revolution particularly in the decade after the war with Iraq. More recently, the cost of living has risen dramatically and young people tend to delay their marriage until they get a salaried job to be able to afford the high living costs.

Decomposition of Change in the Total Fertility Rate

In Iran, childbearing outside marriage forms no part of the cultural tradition and ex-nuptial births can safely be excluded from the current analysis. Overall fertility is, therefore, determined almost exclusively by the proportion of women married and by fertility within marriage. In what follows, we will decompose changes in the total fertility rate into components due to marriage and marital fertility. The results for the national level are presented first, and provincial and rural and urban differences are then discussed.

Table 5.4 shows the decomposition of the change in the total fertility rate for Iran as a whole during the periods 1976–1986, 1986–1996, and 1996–2006 and for rural and urban areas during the periods, 1986–1996 and 1996–2006.

Table 5.4 Decomposition of the change in total fertility rate, 1976–1986, 1986–1996, and 1996–2006, Iran by rural and urban areas (Statistical Centre of Iran, the own-children data from the 1986, 1996 and 2006 censuses, and published data for the census years)

Total	Age group							
Iran 1976–1986	All ages	15–19	20–24	25–29	30–34	35–39	40–44	45–49
Marital fertility	0.22	−0.04	−0.06	0.10	0.09	0.10	0.04	−0.01
Nuptiality	−0.07	−0.02	0.02	−0.04	−0.02	−0.01	0.00	0.00
Total	0.15	−0.06	−0.02	0.06	0.06	0.09	0.03	−0.01
	TFR increased by 0.15 from 6.09 to 6.23							
Iran 1986–1996								
Marital fertility	−3.11	−0.24	−0.40	−0.66	−0.74	−0.63	−0.36	−0.08
Nuptiality	−0.60	−0.25	−0.28	−0.06	0.01	0.00	0.00	0.00
Total	−3.71	−0.49	−0.68	−0.72	−0.75	−0.64	−0.36	−0.08
	TFR declined by 3.70 from 6.23 to 2.52							
Iran 1996–2006								
Marital fertility	−0.42	−0.05	−0.12	−0.07	−0.03	−0.06	−0.06	−0.03
Nuptiality	−0.22	−0.02	−0.10	−0.07	−0.03	−0.01	0.00	0.00
Total	−0.64	−0.07	−0.22	−0.14	−0.06	−0.07	−0.06	−0.03
	TFR decreased by 0.64 from 2.52 to 1.88							
Rural 1986–1996								
Marital fertility	−4.15	−0.29	−0.64	−0.86	−0.95	−0.81	−0.48	−0.11
Nuptiality	−0.72	−0.25	−0.27	−0.13	−0.05	−0.02	−0.01	0.00
Total	−4.87	−0.54	−0.91	−0.99	−0.99	−0.83	−0.49	−0.11
	TFR declined by 4.87 from 7.76 to 2.89							
Rural 1996–2006								
Marital fertility	−0.58	−0.07	−0.14	−0.08	−0.05	−0.12	−0.09	−0.03
Nuptiality	−0.23	0.00	−0.07	−0.09	−0.05	−0.02	0.00	0.00
Total	−0.81	−0.07	−0.21	−0.17	−0.10	−0.14	−0.09	−0.03
	TFR declined by 0.81 from 2.89 to 2.08							
Urban 1986–1996								
Marital fertility	−2.47	−0.13	−0.42	−0.52	−0.58	−0.50	−0.26	−0.05
Nuptiality	−0.47	−0.28	−0.16	−0.03	−0.01	0.00	0.00	0.00
Total	−2.95	−0.41	−0.58	−0.56	−0.59	−0.50	−0.26	−0.05
	TFR declined by 2.95 from 5.19 to 2.24							
Urban 1996–2006								
Marital fertility	−0.26	−0.06	−0.13	−0.04	0.02	−0.01	−0.03	−0.01
Nuptiality	−0.20	−0.02	−0.10	−0.06	−0.02	0.00	0.00	0.00
Total	−0.46	−0.08	−0.23	−0.10	0.00	−0.01	−0.03	−0.01
	TFR declined by 0.46 from 2.24 to 1.78							

1976–1986

As can be seen, total fertility increased by 0.15, from 6.09 in 1976 to 6.23 in 1986. The increase was mainly due to the increase in marital fertility (0.22), but was slightly offset by nuptiality, that is, later age at marriage (−0.07).

The nuptiality component is broken down further by age. Changes in nuptiality tended to reduce the TFR in ages 15–39 but the effect was greater in age group 25–29 than in other age groups. This occurred because the decline in the proportion married was greater in age group 25–29. As discussed earlier, the proportion of married women decreased slightly in all age groups during 1976–1986, except for age group 20–24.

The marital fertility component is also broken down further by age. Changes in marital fertility at younger reproductive ages, 15–19 and 20–24, reduced the TFR whereas changes in other age groups increased the TFR. The decline in marital fertility at earlier ages may be due to the rise of female education during the period. The female literacy rate increased from 35% to 52% during the period. The contribution of marital fertility to the increase in total fertility was about the same across the age groups, 25–29 to 35–39.

1986–1996

The total fertility rate fell by 3.71, from 6.23 in 1986 to 2.52 in 1996. The fall was mainly due to the decline in marital fertility (3.11) with a further decline by 0.60 through nuptiality change. In other words, 84% of the fertility decline was due to the change in marital fertility and only 16% due to nuptiality change.

Changes in nuptiality tended to reduce the TFR in the younger reproductive ages, 15–19, 20–24 and 25–29. This is consistent with the sharp rise in age at marriage during the period which only affects proportions married at the younger ages.

Marital fertility declined in all ages so that the contribution of marital fertility to the change in the TFR was negative in all ages. However, the declines in marital fertility in the middle age groups, 25–29, 30–34, 35–39, were the most pronounced. The decline in marital fertility in younger ages is probably due to delays in the onset of childbearing for young couples whereas the decline in middle and older ages stems from cessation of childbearing at lower parities (see Chapter 4).

1996–2006

The total fertility rate fell by 0.64, from 2.52 in 1996 to 1.88 in 2006. The fall was mainly due to the decline in marital fertility (0.42) with a further decline by 0.22 through nuptiality change. In other words, around 65% of the fertility decline was due to the change in marital fertility and 35% due to nuptiality change, a change from the earlier periods in which the contribution of nuptiality was around 15%.

Changes in nuptiality tended to reduce the TFR in the younger reproductive ages, 20–24, 25–29 and 15–19, respectively. Marital fertility declined in all ages so that the contribution of marital fertility to the change in the TFR was negative in all ages. However, the declines in marital fertility in age groups, 24–29 and 25–29 were the most pronounced. As a whole, the proportion of fertility decline during the recent decade was much lower than the earlier period, but the contribution of marriage to the decline increased substantially during the last period.

Table 5.2 shows that the increase in age at first marriage was somewhat greater in urban areas than in rural areas. However, the decomposition of the change in TFR for both rural and urban areas during the two later periods is identical to that of the total population (Table 5.4). In both areas, the effects of marital fertility on the decline were far greater than those of nuptiality. As expected, during 1986–1996, in both rural and urban areas the effect of nuptiality on fertility was concentrated at younger ages. However, in rural areas the effect of nuptiality was greater in age group 25–29 followed by age group 15–19 while in urban areas the effect in age group 15–19 was greater than in other groups. As for the total population, marital fertility tended to decrease TFR sharply in all age groups in both areas with the largest impact being in the middle ages, 25–39. During 1996–2006, the contribution of nuptiality in both rural and urban areas to the decline of fertility increased substantially, but the share of nuptiality in urban areas (35%) was higher than that of rural areas (28%).

In summary, fertility increased slightly during the first period mainly due to the increase in marital fertility rates. This may stem from the abolition of the family planning program and the lowered level of contraceptive use among families. The socio-cultural context of the post-revolutionary era was another factor in encouraging couples to have more children and higher fertility. However, there was a sharp decline in fertility between 1986 and 1996. In this period, changes in nuptiality reduced fertility by only 15% for the nation as a whole and in both urban and rural areas whereas marital fertility contributed substantially to the fertility decline. In the recent decade, however, the contribution of marriage change at the national level increased to around 35%. It would not be surprising to see the relative impact of nuptiality increasing even more in the future as the scope for change in nuptiality is greater than the scope for change in marital fertility.

Provincial Differences

Table 5.5 shows the changes in TFR and the effects of the two components for the periods 1976–1986, 1986–1996 and 1996–2006 for all provinces. In the first period, the results are quite variable across provinces with six provinces recording falls in the TFR, eight having rises between 0.0 and 0.5, nine having rises between 0.5 and 1.0 and one (Sistan and Baluchistan) having a large rise of 1.77.

Table 5.5 Changes in TFR and the effects of components changes for the periods 1976–86, 1986–96 and 1996–2006, Iran by province (see Table 5.4)

	1976–1986			1986–1996			1996–2006		
	Change	Attributable to:		Change	Attributable to:		Change	Attributable to:	
Province	of TFR	Marriage	Marital fertility	of TFR	Marriage	Marital fertility	of TFR	Marriage	Marital fertility
Iran	0.15	–0.20	0.35	–3.70	–0.50	–3.20	–0.64	–0.23	–0.41
Azarbayjan E	–0.72	–0.34	–0.38	–3.86	–0.57	–3.29	–1.30	–0.18	–1.12
Azarbayjanw	–0.18	–0.32	0.14	–3.31	–0.44	–2.87	–1.41	–0.24	–1.17
Booshehr	0.52	0.05	0.47	–4.47	–0.90	–3.57	–1.03	–0.08	–0.95
Charmahal	0.24	–0.21	0.45	–5.19	–0.84	–4.35	–1.29	–0.49	–0.80
Fars	0.71	–0.12	0.83	–4.29	–0.67	–3.62	–1.33	–0.31	–1.02
Gilan	–0.79	–0.04	–0.75	–2.84	–0.50	–2.34	–0.89	–0.10	–0.79
Hamadan	0.24	–0.13	0.37	–4.48	–0.73	–3.75	–1.60	–0.30	–1.30
Hormozgan	0.79	0.27	0.52	–4.13	–1.07	–3.06	–1.07	–0.32	–0.75
Ilam	0.46	–0.24	0.70	–5.05	–1.29	–3.76	–1.90	–0.55	–1.35
Isfahan	–0.10	–0.15	0.05	–3.68	–0.55	–3.13	–0.66	–0.29	–0.37
Kerman	0.32	–0.06	0.38	–4.24	–0.85	–3.39	–1.22	–0.26	–0.96
Kermanshah	0.40	–0.23	0.63	–3.88	–0.61	–3.27	–1.42	–0.32	–1.10
Khorasan[a]	0.42	0.01	0.41	–3.89	–0.62	–3.27	–1.56	–0.20	–1.36
Khoozestan	0.90	0.10	0.80	–4.28	–0.74	–3.54	–1.61	–0.55	–1.06
Kohgilooyeh	0.68	–0.12	0.80	–5.54	–1.07	–4.47	–1.51	–0.69	–0.82
Kurdistan	0.50	–0.02	0.52	–4.31	–0.57	–3.74	–1.68	–0.29	–1.39
Lorestan	0.38	–0.38	0.76	–4.61	–0.95	–3.66	–1.93	–0.49	–1.44
Markazi	–0.04	0.05	–0.09	–3.96	–0.54	–3.42	–1.00	–0.05	–0.96
Mazandaran	–0.17	–0.22	0.05	–3.21	–0.49	–2.72	–1.11	–0.09	–1.02
Semnan	0.58	0.07	0.51	–3.06	–0.50	–2.56	–0.72	–0.20	–0.52
Sistan and Baluchistan	1.77	–0.12	1.89	–4.76	–0.65	–4.11	–1.15	–0.48	–0.67
Tehran	0.58	–0.20	0.78	–2.71	–0.38	–2.33	–0.69	–0.25	–0.44
Yazd	0.82	0.27	0.55	–3.54	–0.72	–2.82	–0.79	–0.26	–0.53
Zanjan	0.25	–0.46	0.71	–4.40	–0.75	–3.65	–1.44	–0.34	–1.10

[a] By 2006 Khorasan province was divided into three provinces (South, North and Razavi), and thus the result for Khorasan province in 2006 is an average of the three provinces. Three other provinces of Qom, Gazvin, and Golestan were added to the provinces in 2006 but due to the lack of data in earlier periods it was not possible to get the results for the periods.

However, marital fertility fell in only three provinces in this period. Thus, the national rise in marital fertility, attributed to a fall off in the family planning programme, was evident in almost all provinces of the country. On the other hand, in seven of the 24 provinces, in contrast to the national trend, nuptiality change had a positive effect on the TFR. These were provinces in which the revolutionary government's incentives to marry early presumably had a larger impact.

In the second period, 1986–1996, there was a highly consistent picture across provinces with all provinces experiencing considerable falls in TFR and in all provinces the effects on TFR of nuptiality and martial fertility change were negative, with the effects of marital fertility being much greater than the effects of nuptiality. In general, between 14% and 20% of the fertility change in this period was due to the change in age at marriage. Similar to the second period, both nuptiality and marital fertility had a negative impact on fertility during the third period, 1996–2006. However, various patterns emerged during this period. In the majority of provinces (15), between 20% and 46% of the decline in fertility was due to nuptiality. This category consisted of provinces that had lower mean age at marriage in earlier periods, and thus, there was a change in the age at marriage during the later period. In six provinces, the contribution of nuptiality to marriage change was around 11–19%, and only in three provinces nuptiality had a negative impact on fertility change between 5% and 8%. These two categories were composed of provinces that had lower fertility and relatively higher age at marriage during the latter two periods.

Discussion

The results of the decomposition analysis have shown that changes in fertility were mainly attributable to falls in marital fertility during each of the periods examined. In this regard, the Iranian fertility transition is more like the early fertility transition in Indonesia than the transitions in East Asian countries (Casterline 1991; Retherford and Ogawa 1978; Ogawa, and Retherford 1993; Jones 1997, 2007; Jones et al. 2009). Studies suggest that the impact of change of marriage patterns on Indonesian fertility is also rising (Hull 2003). The reduction in Iran's marital fertility was four times more important than changes in marriage patterns in Iran as a whole and in all provinces and urban and rural areas. Around 85% of the decline in fertility was due to the decrease in marital fertility during the period 1986–1996; nuptiality was responsible for only 15% of the decline. While during the third period, 1996–2006, around 35% of the decline was due to nuptiality. This was confirmed by Erfani and McQuillan (2008) who found that marriage has contributed around 31 percent of the fertility decline. This indicates that Iranian women have controlled their fertility within marriage. The means of fertility control that they have used are considered in Chapters 6 and 7.

The analysis in this chapter underlines the point made in Chapter 3 that the pattern of fertility decline after 1986 was similar in all regions of the country and in both urban and rural areas. The story of fertility decline in Iran is, therefore, a national story not a complex of stories of differences across provinces.

References

Abbasi-Shavazi MJ (2000) Effects of marital fertility and nuptiality on fertility transition in the Islamic Republic of Iran. Working Papers in Demography, No. 84. The Australian National University, Canberra

Aghajanian A (1998) Family and family change in Iran. In: Hennon CB, Brubaker TH (eds) Diversity in families: a global perspective. Wadsworth Publishing Company, New York

Azimi H (1981) Population growth and its needs. Budget and Planning Organization (Persian). Department of Human Resources and Social Planning, Tehran

Bahramitash R, Kazemipour S (2006) Myths and realities of the impact of Islam on women: Changing martial status in Iran. Critique: Crit Middle Eastern Stud 15(3):111–128

Casterline JB (1991) Fertility transition in Asia, Presented at the International Union for the Scientific Study of Population [IUSSP] Committee on Comparative Analysis of Fertility and University of Zimbabwe Seminar on the Course of Fertility Transition in Sub-Saharan Africa, Harare, Zimbabwe, 19–22 November 1991

Erfani A, McQuillan K (2008) Rapid fertility decline in Iran: Analysis of intermediate variables, Journal of Biosocial Sciences 40(3):459–478

Hull TH (2003) Demographic perspectives on the future of Indonesian family. J Popul Res 20(1):51–66

Jones GW (2007) Delayed marriage and very low fertility in Pacific Asia. Popul Dev Rev 33(3):453–478

Jones GW (1997) The demise of universal marriage in east and South-east Asia. In: Jones GW, Douglas R, Caldwell JC, D'Souza RM (eds) The continuing demographic transition. Clarendon Press, Oxford, pp 51–79

Jones GW, Straughan PT, Chan A (eds) (2009) Ultra-low fertility in Pacific Asia: trends, causes and policy issues. Rutledge, London

Kitagawa EM (1955) Components of a difference between two rates. J Am Stat Assoc 50:1168–1194

Knodel J (1983) Natural fertility: age patterns, levels, and trends. In: Rodolfo A. Bulatao, Ronald D. Lee (eds) Determinants of fertility in developing countries. Academic, New York, pp 61–102

McNicoll G, Singarimbun M (1981) Fertility decline in Indonesia: analysis and interpretation. National Academic Press, Washington D.C

Mehryar AH, Tajdini F (1998) Population and development in the Islamic Republic of Iran: a review of the main findings of the 1996 census and other sources of data. Institute for Research on Planning and Development, Tehran

Ogawa N, Retherford R (1993) The resumption of fertility decline in Japan: 1972–1992. Popul Dev Rev 19(4):703–741

Retherford RD, Ogawa N (1978) Decomposition of the change in the total fertility rate in the Republic of Korea, 1966–70. Social Biol 25(2):115–127

Smith P (1983) The impact of age at marriage and proportion marrying on fertility. In Rodolfo A. Bulatao, Ronald D. Lee (eds) Determinats of fertility in developing countries. Academic Press, New York, pp. 473–531

Statistical Center of Iran (2007) Results of the 2006 Census: selected tables. Statistical Center of Iran, Tehran

VandenHeuvel A, McDonald P (1994) Marriage and divorce. In: Lucas D, Meyer P (eds) Beginning population studies. Australian National University, Canberra, pp 69–90

Chapter 6
Contraceptive Use: Trends, Levels and Correlates*

Introduction

Iran, along with other Muslim countries, Indonesia, Pakistan, Tunisia, Egypt, and Turkey, officially adopted a population policy in the 1960s to reduce population growth by implementing family planning (Nortman and Hofstatter 1978). The first general family planning clinic was established in 1968 in Tehran (Ministry of Health 2003). By 1976, the Iran Fertility Survey showed that 26% of married women aged 15–49 were using a modern method of contraception (Aghajanian 1994).

The official family planning program was suspended after the Islamic Revolution, however, the Ministry of Health clinics never completely stopped providing family planning services to clients. In 1980, the Minister of Health received a ruling in answer to his question about the legitimacy of birth control in the form of an edict issued by Imam Khomeini indicating that Islam permits the use of contraception (Ministry of Health 2003). In 1989, the family planning program was revived with massive financial and policy support from the government and religious leaders. Since 1989, the family planning program has received an annual centralized budget and all services remain free of charge through the public sector. The information, education and communication (IEC) component of Iran's family planning services has been strongly and continuously implemented throughout the country.

The religious ideology of Islam is said to favour birth-control policy depending on the government's position, that is, different governments interpret the rules of Islam differently (Omran 1992). Iran is a good example of this as, after the revolution in 1979, a pronatalist policy used Islam's rules in order to encourage people to have more children and increase fertility, while an antinatalist viewpoint in the late 1980s applied Islam's rules to legitimate birth-control policy and contraceptive use. However, Imam Khomeini, the religious leader of the Islamic Revolution, never prohibited the use of contraception. Rather, it was the war with Iraq in 1980 that led to the neglect of the family planning program as well as to the encouragement of early marriage and high fertility (Mehryar 2005). After the revival of the family planning program in 1989,

---

*This chapter is drawn from Hosseini-Chavoshi (2007).

M.J. Abbasi-Shavazi et al., *The Fertility Transition in Iran: Revolution and Reproduction*,

sterilization was added to the list of family planning services provided by the government sector. In 1993, DMPA and Norplant were also added to the program.

This chapter first presents a brief review of trends in the prevalence of contraceptive practice among married women. Second, the profile of contraceptive users and non-users is investigated, and then unmet need for contraception and reasons for non-use are discussed for married women as a whole and specifically for married women in the four selected low fertility provinces. The patterns of contraceptive method mix are described as are the sources of contraceptives among users. Finally, contraceptive practice is examined in terms of different socio-demographic factors.

Data and Analytical Methods

The 2000 Iran Demographic and Health Survey (IDHS) is used to investigate contraceptive use and its determinants at the national and provincial levels. Specific attention is also given to the provinces targeted in the 2002 Iran Fertility Transition Survey (IFTS) and the 2005 Iran Low Fertility Survey (ILFS). An important difference between these data sets is that the ILFS data allow investigation of women's current contraceptive use according to their intentions, that is, whether they are attempting to have no more births or are spacing births.

Data from KAP (knowledge, attitudes and practice) surveys conducted between 1994 and 1997 as well as secondary published data from the 1976 Iran Fertility Survey (IFS) and the 1989, 1991, and 1992 KAP surveys are used to show trends in contraceptive use over the last two decades. The 1976 Iran Fertility Survey and the 1989 KAP survey collected nationally representative data about fertility and family planning, while all other surveys conducted since 1971 collected provincially representative data about fertility and family planning. The sample sizes of the data sets used in this chapter are large enough to measure the level of contraceptive practice and to examine some determinants associated with contraceptive use at the provincial level.

Current contraceptive prevalence from the IDHS provides only a crude estimator of family planning practice as it refers only to currently married women regardless of whether they were sexually active or not. Respondents were not asked about their sexual activity or sexual practices, for example, some women who have undergone sterilization or are using an IUD may be sexually inactive, or may be infecund. Also, in the case of women using more than one method simultaneously, for example, a traditional method with condom, only the most effective method was recorded regardless of whether it was the dominant method or not. The 2005 ILFS includes information about the respondent's 'contraceptive history' in the four selected low fertility provinces. The contraceptive use history spans the full reproductive life of each respondent. These data are used especially in Chapter 7 in which a dynamic approach to the analysis of contraceptive use is taken.

A comparison of the 2005 ILFS with the 2000 IDHS indicates a very close correspondence for prevalence of contraception among all women aged 15–49 years. The estimated Contraceptive Prevalence Rate (CPR) for the low fertility provinces in the year 2000 was 56% based on the 2000 IDHS and 57% based on the 2005 ILFS. Further, the contraceptive prevalence trend derived from the ILFS data is very close to that derived from the KAP surveys and the IDHS. The closeness of these results substantiates the quality of data in both the ILFS and in all the data sets used in this research.

Contraceptive Use: Level and Trend

Contraceptive prevalence is one of the main indicators of a family planning program. It measures the cross-sectional level of contraceptive practice among women of reproductive age. As sexual relations in Iran are legally and socially acceptable only within marriage, in all surveys, only currently married women were asked about their contraceptive practice. Therefore, in this chapter, all analysis relates to contraceptive use among currently married women aged 15–49 unless otherwise stated.

The trend in contraceptive use in Iran (Table 6.1) shows that the percentage using any form of contraception among currently married women at ages 15–49 almost doubled from the 1970s to the end of the 1990s. The 1976 IFS revealed that 36% of currently married women aged 15–49 were using any type of contraception. This can be considered as the result of the population policy adopted in 1967 and the first family planning campaign (Agha 1985; Aghajanian 1994). Among the 26% using modern contraceptive methods, about 17% were pill users, 4% condom, while less than 5% of women were using the IUD or any other form of modern

Table 6.1 Contraceptive prevalence rates (%) by method among currently married women aged 15–49, Iran, 1976–2000 (Iran Fertility Survey [Aghajanian 1994] for 1976; the figures for 1989–2000 come from the 1989–1997 KAP surveys and the 2000 IDHS)

	IFS	IKAP	IKAP	IKAP	IKAP	IKAP	IKAP	IKAP	IDHS
Method	1976	1989	1992	1993	1994	1995	1996	1997	2000
Pill	17.3	18.1	22.6	24.5	22.0	22.8	21.9	20.9	18.4
Condom	4.0	5.7	6.4	6.7	6.6	5.7	5.6	5.4	5.9
IUD	1.4	3.7	7.1	7.2	7.8	7.1	8.3	8.3	8.5
Female sterilization			7.6	9.2	11.1	13.7	15.0	15.5	17.1
Male sterilization			0.9	1.0	1.2	1.3	1.6	1.9	2.7
Injectable (DMPA)					0.5	1.3	2.5	2.9	2.8
Norplant					0.0	0.0	0.0	0.5	0.5
Other	3.2	3.0		0.6	1.9	1.7	1.2	0.6	0.1
Traditional	10.1	18.4	20.0	18.6	18.9	19.2	18.0	16.9	17.8
All method	36.0	48.9	64.6	67.8	70.0	72.8	73.7	72.9	73.8
No. of women	4,715	8,975	36,000	40,963	40,995	41,082	41,347	42,645	87,400

contraceptive method available in the private sector. Users of traditional methods with 10% coverage comprised about 28% of contraceptive users. It should be mentioned that traditional method users in Iran mainly use withdrawal and a very low percentage (less than 1% of women) use periodic abstinence.

Prior to the revival of the family planning program, a survey undertaken by the Ministry of Health in Autumn 1989 showed that 49% of currently married Iranian women of reproductive ages were using a contraceptive method (Ministry of Health 1990). The increase between this and previous cross sectional surveys was due to increases in both modern and traditional methods. Whilst the level of use of modern methods increased from 26% to about 30%, the use of traditional methods increased substantially from 10% to 18%. This increase is consistent with the onset of fertility decline from 1984 described in Chapters 3 and 4. The growth in the use of traditional methods relates to the fact that the government did not support the use of modern methods either financially or politically during the 1980s. The relatively high level of usage in the years before the revival of the family planning program indicates a strong desire on the part of couples to control their fertility, a desire not stimulated by government information programs.

The first survey conducted after the revival of the official family planning program in 1989, the 1992 KAP survey, covered 2,000 households in each province of Iran and collected information about contraceptive use among currently married women aged 15–44. The weighted result for the country (Table 6.1) revealed that after less than 3 years of reactivation of the family planning program, contraceptive prevalence had risen to 64.5%. The rise in prevalence between 1989 and 1992 was almost totally in the increased use of modern methods, especially sterilization. Pill users comprised 23% of eligible women and 9% used sterilization methods. The prevalence of IUD use also doubled, reaching 7% of eligible women, and other modern and traditional methods remained almost at the same rates. Between 1993 and 1997, cross sectional surveys with similar sample sizes were conducted at the beginning of each year to evaluate the family planning program in terms of its impact on fertility decline, and to estimate the contraceptive prevalence rate. By 1997, contraceptive users comprised 73% of all eligible women. Around a quarter of women were using the pill and DMPA. About 19% were using traditional methods, a figure unchanged since 1989. The increase in the prevalence rate from 1989 to 1997 (24% points) was due entirely to the increased use of modern methods notably sterilization which accounted for 20 of the 24% points increase.

DMPA was introduced to the family planning service provided by the public sector in 1993. Since then, pill users have been advised to switch from the pill to DMPA as this method was thought to be more effective because women would not have to remember to take a pill every day. Norplant was available in the family planning program for a few years from 1994 to 1997 but due to a high demand for early removal it was no longer provided by the public sector family planning service and is now available only in the private sector. Norplant users never exceeded more than 0.5% of women. Aside from the modern methods mentioned in the table, a small proportion of women used other types of modern methods.

Method Mix Among Contraceptive Users

Figure 6.1 shows that during the 1990s around one-third of contraceptive users were using contraceptive pills. The next most commonly used modern contraceptive was sterilization, followed by IUD, condom, and DMPA. After the re-activation of the family planning program, the proportion of traditional method users among all users slightly decreased from about one-third of users to about one-quarter. This may have been due to the extension of the government program into areas of the country that had low levels of family planning usage. As discussed below, traditional methods are more likely to be used in the more advanced, urban areas (Fig. 6.1).

During the second half of the 1990s, there was only a slight increase in the contraceptive prevalence rate – less than 1%. However, with the increase in sterilization and DMPA, there was a shift to a more reliable mix of methods. This was probably a result of the activities of the government program in convincing women to adopt more reliable methods.

The use of traditional methods consists almost entirely of withdrawal. Periodic abstinence is not generally used as a main method but as a secondary or backup method, and probably those women who use periodic abstinence as a backup to withdrawal, are more successful than those who use withdrawal only. Withdrawal or coitus interruptus is one of the oldest documented methods of avoiding pregnancy among Muslims. The method is recorded under the name of '*Nazdiki-e monghata*'

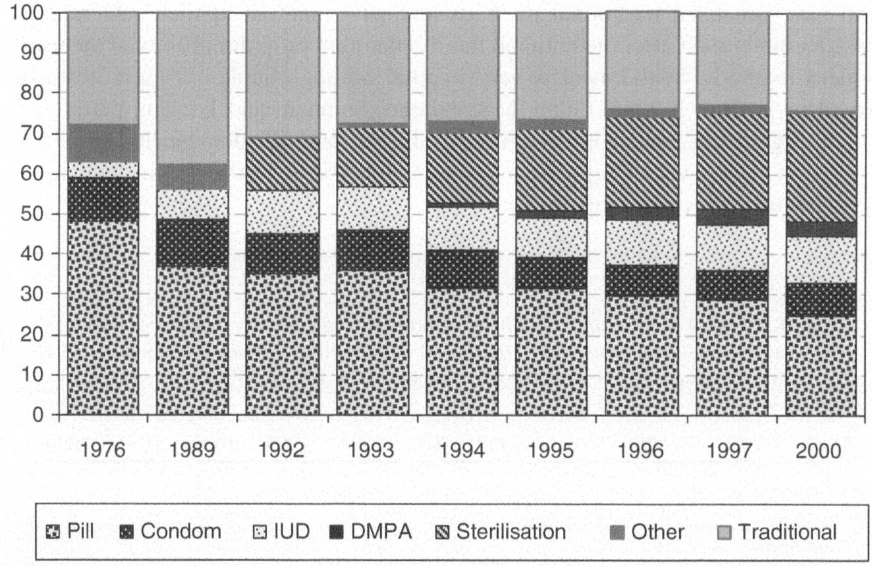

Fig. 6.1 Percentage distribution of contraceptive users by method, Iran, 1976–2000 (Iran Fertility Survey [Aghajanian 1994] for 1976; the figures for 1989–2000 come from the 1989–1997 KAP surveys and the 2000 IDHS)

or '*Azl*' in Persian references, and its legitimacy has been recorded in principal references of Islam such as the '*Hadith*' (tenets of Islamic guidance spoken by the Prophet Mohammad and recorded by his disciples/followers, Omran 1992). Withdrawal is also considered to be a male-initiated method, demonstrating male participation in family planning (Karra et al. 1997; Gribble 2003). However, this is a method that requires both male and female participation, and women can be actively involved. For example, Mehryar (2005), quoting from the famous Persian Sufi poet Jalaladin Molavi Rumi (AD 1207–1273), narrates the story of a merchant advising his daughter how to avoid pregnancy by using withdrawal as a method.

There is no information during the implementation of the first family planning program in the 1970s that shows to what extent this method was used by couples at that time. The 1976 IFS showed that women in urban areas were much more likely to be practising a contraceptive method to avoid pregnancy as their counterparts in rural areas (54% versus 20%), and the proportion of withdrawal users among contraceptive users was four times as high among urban residents as rural residents (Aghajanian and Mehryar 1999). Successive surveys also showed (Table 6.2) that, in urban areas, around one third of family planning users during the decade of the 1990s were withdrawal users. Further, the prevalence of withdrawal among users remained about 1.5 times more likely in urban areas than in rural areas. However, it is interesting to note that the proportion of married women using withdrawal remained at roughly the same level in both urban and rural areas from the time that the family planning program commenced while the frequency of modern method use increased substantially. This suggests that there has always been a sub-group who have practised traditional methods and who maintained their adherence to these methods even after the national family planning program promoted the use of modern methods. Withdrawal is very popular among couples in more advanced provinces such as Tehran, Gilan, Mazandaran, Semnan, and Isfahan, particularly among highly educated couples (Abbasi-Shavazi and Khademzadeh 2004). This usage may have a very long history. Interestingly, these are the provinces that now have the lowest levels of fertility.

Table 6.2 Use of modern and traditional methods among currently married women aged 15–49, urban and rural areas, Iran, 1976–2000 (Iran Fertility Survey [Aghajanian 1994] for 1976; the figures for 1989–2000 come from the 1989–1997 KAP surveys and the 2000 IDHS)

Region/method	1976	1989	1992	1993	1994	1995	1996	1997	2000
Urban									
Modern	34	37	47	52	53	53	55	56	55
Traditional	20	27	27	25	25	26	24	22	22
Rural									
Modern	15	23	41	45	49	54	57	58	57
Traditional	5	8	10	10	10	10	10	9	10

Table 6.3 Percentage of currently married women aged 15–49 using different methods of contraception, urban and rural areas, Iran, 2000 (The 2000 Iran Demographic and Health Survey)

Area of residence	Contraceptive method use								Number of women
	Any method	Sterilization Female	Sterilization Male	IUD	DMPA	Pill	Condom	Withdrawal	
Rural	67.2	19.0	1.3	5.5	5.6	21.8	3.5	9.6	42,514
Urban	77.1	16.2	3.4	10.0	1.4	16.6	7.2	21.4	44,886
Total	73.7	17.2	2.7	8.4	2.8	18.5	5.9	17.2	87,400

In 2000, the coverage of IUD was almost double in urban areas (Table 6.3). Women in urban areas have greater access to IUD insertion through the private and public sectors. Government health centres throughout urban areas offer professional facilities for IUD insertion and provision of follow-up services for users. Additionally, the private sector is active in IUD insertion for women particularly through physicians and gynecologists. Private sector midwives and physicians are concentrated in urban areas and the government has encouraged private sector activity in the area of IUD services by offering subsidised access to IUDs to this sector.

Government policy also responded to a preference by many women in urban areas, particularly professional and middle class women, for using the services of the private sector. Professional women particularly preferred the 'out of hours' services offered by the private sector. Government policy has encouraged participation by the private sector in professional delivery of family planning services. Offered financial encouragement to provide IUD services, the private sector which was already equipped in terms of human resources, recommended IUD insertion to women seeking contraception. With this arrangement, the private sector benefited and so too did the government through private delivery of a cost efficient and long-term method.

Health houses located in rural areas at the village level are not professionally equipped to offer IUD insertion services to women. As a result, women who seek IUDs are referred by health houses to rural health centres that are located in larger villages. This reduces rural women's access to IUDs as women may be reluctant to travel to a distant health centre. Instead, women may take up a method such as the pill or condom provided by the nearby health house. This problem of access has resulted in greater distribution of the contraceptive pill in rural areas than urban areas. On the other hand, female sterilization is used a little more in rural areas than urban areas indicating that travel away from the home village is not an obstacle for women in rural areas who wish to end their childbearing.

DMPA was introduced to the health network system in the early 1990s. It is a temporary method requiring monthly injections for a period of 3 months. The government promoted this method as it was a more cost effective method than the contraceptive pill. DMPA has easier follow-up, less risk of use failure, and less risk of method failure. As a result of rural health house promotion of DMPA, its prevalence rate increased markedly in rural areas, but not in urban areas.

Socio-Demographic Differentials in Contraceptive Use

Levels and patterns of contraceptive use vary among couples and women with different social and demographic characteristics both in developing (Tuladhar 1985; Mahmud and Islam 1995; Varena et al. 1996; Koc 2000; Lutalo et al. 2000; Balaiah et al. 2005) and developed countries (Lavecchia et al. 1986; Ringheim 1997; Oddens and Lehert 1997). Moreover, women with similar demographic characteristics practise different patterns of birth control behaviour within different social classifications and areas of residence (Mosher and Bachrach 1986; Svare et al. 1997; Degraff et al. 1997). Such variations have also been studied among Iranian women, and the primary social demographic characteristics such as education, number of children and place of residence were found to be associated with contraceptive use (Malekafzali 1992; Aghajanian 1994; Ministry of Health 2002; Abbasi-Shavazi et al. 2004). With the exception of education, recent studies show some convergence of reproductive and fertility control behaviour of women in different social and demographic backgrounds such as area of residence or age groups (Hosseini-Chavoshi et al. 2004; Abbasi-Shavazi et al. 2004).

Using the 2000 IDHS data set, differentials in contraceptive use are first investigated at the regional level. Second, due to lack of information on cultural factors in the IDHS data, the 2002 IFTS is used to show contraceptive differentials according to ethnicity and religion. Third, the variation according to place of residence is analysed with particular attention to the four selected low fertility provinces. Finally, all social and demographic factors are examined together to explore the association of each component when other factors are held constant. It is hypothesised that women who are more educated or are employed or are living in the cities will be more likely to use contraception to avoid pregnancy.

Region of Residence

For regional comparison and further analysis related to the impact of place of residence, provinces are categorised into eight groups based on geographic units sharing religious and cultural characteristics. Provinces in the north of Iran (Gilan and Mazandaran) and Tehran City are categorised as a single entity 'North + Tehran City' as they share equally very low levels of fertility and high levels of women's autonomy (Hosseini-Chavoshi et al. 2004). Provinces located in the central area of Iran are given two categories. The first category is 'Central' where the majority of people are Persian speaking ethnic Fars (provinces of Fars, Hamedan, Isfahan, Markazi, Qazvin, Qom, Semnan, Yazd, and Tehran province outside Tehran City). The second category comprises people who are mainly ethnic Lor (provinces of Chaharmahal, Kohogiluyeh and Lorestan). North-western provinces of the country are categorised 'North West, Turk' and represent Turkish speaking ethnic Turks of whom a considerable percentage are Sunni (provinces of Ardebil, East and West

Azarbaijan and Zanjan). Western provinces in Iran are categorised as 'West, Kurd' and represent predominantly Sunni ethnic Kurds (provinces of Ilam, Kermanshah, and Kordestan).

Provinces in the south and southwest are categorised 'South and South West' and share some cultural characteristics with neighbouring Arabian countries in the Persian Gulf (provinces of Booshehr, Hormozgan, and Khuzestan). The category 'East and North East' includes the provinces of Golestan, Kerman, and Khorasan and comprises substantial rural areas. This category comprises people who demonstrate cultural characteristics similar to peoples from Afghanistan. The last category comprises the single province of Sistan and Baluchistan and is characterised by the country's highest level of fertility. This population is predominantly ethnic Baluch who are Sunni.

The results in Table 6.4 show that the provinces with ethnic minorities (Turk, Kurd, Lor) follow almost the same pattern in contraceptive use in terms of type of method. Couples in these regions prefer to use modern methods of contraception rather than traditional methods. The North (27%) and the Central Fars (19%) regions have the highest percentages using traditional methods. They also have the highest rate of users of all the regions. In contrast, women in the West and North West regions have the highest level of usage of temporary modern methods. The West Kurd and Central Lor regions had the highest levels of usage of sterilization.

Table 6.4 Percentage of currently married women aged 15–49 using different methods of contraception by region of residence, Iran, 2000 (The 2000 Iran Demographic and Health Survey)

Region of residence	Contraceptive method use									Number of women
	Any method	Sterilization		IUD	DMPA	Pill	Condom	Withdrawal		
		Female	Male							
Iran	73.7	17.2	2.7	8.4	2.8	18.5	5.9	17.2		87,400
North and Tehran City	79.5	15.7	3.7	10.4	1.0	15.2	5.8	26.9		7,368
Central, majority Fars	76.7	18.5	4.2	9.0	2.3	15.8	7.1	19.1		26,549
West, majority Kurd	75.1	22.7	1.2	8.6	5.6	24.3	4.3	6.5		9,274
Central, majority Lor	71.2	22.9	1.8	6.8	4.5	22.6	4.2	7.5		9,676
North-west, majority Turk	72.8	16.1	1.2	11.1	5.3	22.8	3.9	11.1		12,512
South and South-west	66.4	15.7	1.2	4.8	2.7	23.3	6.6	11.4		9,932
East and North-east	69.1	16.5	1.5	5.5	2.8	18.5	6.4	17.2		8,783
Sistan and Baluchistan	41.4	5.8	0.3	2.1	4.6	19.6	3.2	3.8		3,306

However, as was discussed in Chapter 3, these provinces are not characterised by low fertility, and the choice of sterilization is undertaken when women already have a relatively high number of children. Women from Lorestan chose sterilization methods (rarely vasectomy) only after reaching a high number of children, and only 7% practised traditional methods, indicating low male acceptance of birth control.

Almost one-third of women in the South and South West and in the East and North East were not using any contraception at the time of the 2000 survey. Using modern contraceptive methods is more prevalent among women in the south, and traditional methods are more common in the east. The contraceptive use pattern in Sistan and Baluchistan is strikingly different compared to other regions; 59% of women were not using any type of contraception at the time of the survey. Only 6% of women had limited their child bearing by undergoing sterilization (rarely vasectomy), and almost the same figure (4%) were using a traditional method. The contraceptive pill was the main method used in this province.

In all regions, withdrawal was much more likely to be used in urban areas than in rural areas. The urban areas in the North and Tehran City region had an extraordinarily high level of contraceptive prevalence but the lowest use of sterilization of all of the regions other than Sistan and Baluchistan. In sum, the use of withdrawal is associated with the lowest levels of fertility while the usage of sterilization is associated with somewhat higher levels of fertility. Overall, the differences in methods mix between regions and the overall high usage rates point to a capacity of the national family planning program to adapt its delivery to local preferences. Flexibility is thus a mark of its success.

Ethnicity and Religion

The 2002 IFTS was conducted in the four selected provinces of Sistan and Baluchistan, West Azarbaijan, Gilan and Yazd (Abbasi-Shavazi et al. 2004). Different patterns of contraceptive use by language (ethnic) group were observed. Sterilization levels were relatively similar across all ethnic groups with the exception of the Baluch who had a very low usage of sterilization. Kurds, Turks and Baluch (given their lower use overall) had relatively high levels of use of the hormonal methods, the pill and DMPA (Table 6.5).

The highest levels of pill use were among Kurds, Turks and Gilak women. In addition, Baluchi and Kurdish women were more likely to use DMPA than other groups. Gilak and Baluch women were less likely to use IUD and Norplant (methods with low failure rates at least during the first 5 years). Baluchi women are probably not using these methods due to inaccessibility or due to their relatively high demand for more children. These reasons do not apply to Gilak women, and further studies are needed to investigate specifically the low prevalence of IUD and Norplant on the one hand and the high prevalence of traditional methods on the other hand among Gilak women. Distinct patterns for Turk and Fars women were the high use of IUD for Turks and condoms by Fars. The pattern of contraceptive use among Sunni women

Table 6.5 Percentage using different methods of contraception by ethnicity and religion, four selected provinces, 2002 (The 2002 Iran Fertility Transition Survey)

	Type of contraception						
Place of residence, ethnicity and religion	Sterilization	IUD, Norplant	DMPA	Pill	Condom	Withdrawal	Number of women
Ethnicity							
Fars	20.1	8.8	1.0	16.8	11.1	21.0	1,581
Turk	21.0	13.1	4.5	23.6	3.7	15.3	868
Gilak	18.8	2.9	1.5	23.1	5.6	27.1	1,010
Kurd	23.3	8.7	9.4	26.5	1.9	7.0	567
Baluch	4.0	0.7	8.8	18.0	2.5	1.7	830
Religion							
Shiite	20.3	7.7	2.4	20.6	6.5	21.7	3,465
Sunni	13.5	4.7	8.8	24.3	2.2	4.9	1,522
Religion and region							
Shiite, Sistan	14.5	5.5	3.4	29.0	6.9	9.5	402
Sunni, Sistan	4.1	0.8	8.8	18.4	2.6	1.7	837
Shiite, other 3 provinces	20.8	7.9	2.3	19.8	6.4	22.9	3,063
Sunni, other 3 provinces	21.2	8.0	8.9	29.0	2.0	7.5	685
Total	18.2	6.8	4.3	21.7	5.2	16.6	4,987

in Sistan and Baluchistan is similar to that already described for Baluchi-speaking women. Fars and Gilak women used condoms and traditional methods much more commonly compared with other groups. Finally, Gilak women (with high overall use) had a low usage of the IUD while Turks had a high level of usage.

By religion, around 60% of Sunni women and around 80% of Shiite women were using contraception at the time of the survey in April 2002. The overall level of use of modern methods was similar for the two groups of women but the use of traditional methods was four times higher for Shiite women than for Sunni women. Within the modern methods, the method mix also varied between Sunni and Shiite women. Sunni women were much more likely than Shiite women to use hormonal methods while Shiite women were more likely to use sterilization, IUDs and condoms.

When Sunni and Shiite women residing in Yazd, Gilan and West Azarbaijan are compared, the main difference is the heavy use of hormonal methods by the Sunni women offset by the heavy use of withdrawal by the Shiite women.

In Sistan and Baluchistan, Shiite women have a pattern of usage that is more similar to the Sunni women in Yazd, Gilan and West Azarbaijan than to Shiite women in these provinces, with a strong emphasis on hormonal methods. This could indicate a heavier impact of the government program in the mainly rural and distant province of Sistan and Baluchistan. Sunni women in Sistan and Baluchistan (essentially the Baluch) have by far the lowest overall prevalence rate at 34%. Where a method is used, the hormonal methods dominate again probably indicating the impact of the government program.

Given the high degree of overlap of ethnicity, religion and province, the impacts of any one of these three variables upon contraceptive usage is difficult to isolate.

The Age of the Woman

Contraceptive usage is relatively high even as young as ages 15–19 with close to 40% of married women at this age using any method. Usage of any method then rises with age reaching a peak in age group 35–39 when only 14% of women are not using contraception. Sterilization is uncommon under age 30 but rises from age 30 to reach a peak of 41% by age group 40–44. This is a remarkably high level of sterilization by any international standard. The use of hormonal methods is near its peak as early as age group 20–24. It then peaks in the next age group, 25–29, at almost 30%. Expectedly, the usage of hormonal methods falls off as sterilization rates rise with age. With a lower prevalence level, the age pattern of IUD usage is similar to that of the hormonal methods (Table 6.6).

Condom usage varies little in prevalence across the different age groups, with a prevalence ranging from 5% to 7% across most ages. The use of withdrawal also does not vary very much by age. The use of condoms and withdrawal most likely become regular aspects of the couple's sexual behaviour among those that use these methods.

The Number of Children

The use of sterilization is very limited until women have three children and then its use rises sharply as the number of children rises. Among those with three surviving children, 24% used sterilization compared to 47% among those with five or more children. That sterilization is associated with high fertility supports the observation above that it is more commonly used in regions that have somewhat higher levels

Table 6.6 Percentage of currently married women using different methods of contraception by age group, Iran, 2000 (The 2000 Iran Demographic and Health Survey)

Age group/ area of residence	Contraceptive method use									Number of women
	Any method	Sterilization		IUD	DMPA	Pill	Condom	Withdrawal		
		Female	Male							
15–19	37.4	0.1	0.0	4.2	0.9	14.4	4.9	12.6		6,182
20–24	60.9	0.3	0.4	10.8	3.1	22.3	5.9	17.1		14,052
25–29	74.3	3.7	1.0	13.2	3.8	25.6	7.0	18.9		16,519
30–34	81.6	16.4	3.0	11.1	3.5	21.2	7.0	18.5		15,569
35–39	86.1	30.5	5.4	6.8	3.0	16.3	5.8	17.4		13,570
40–44	83.3	36.5	4.7	4.4	2.4	13.2	4.8	16.4		12,059
45–49	68.3	31.7	3.3	2.2	1.5	8.8	4.3	15.5		9,449

Table 6.7 Percentage of currently married women 15–49 using different methods of contraception, by number of children ever born, Iran, 2000 (The 2000 Iran Demographic and Health Survey)

Number of children	Contraceptive method use								Number of women
	Any method	Sterilization		IUD	DMPA	Pill	Condom	Withdrawal	
		Female	Male						
0	19.5	0.0	0.2	0.1	0.0	3.7	3.1	12.1	11,499
1	74.8	0.2	0.2	13.5	1.9	26.9	8.7	22.4	14,756
2	85.9	3.4	2.7	15.7	3.2	25.5	8.8	25.2	15,398
3	85.3	19.2	4.9	10.3	3.3	19.8	6.9	19.8	11,862
4	85.1	32.4	4.7	6.8	3.4	17.5	5.3	14.4	10,033
5+	80.5	43.1	3.6	2.8	4.3	14.3	2.5	9.1	23,852

Table 6.8 Percentage of currently married women 15–49 using different methods of contraception by level of education, Iran, 2000 (The 2000 Iran Demographic and Health Survey)

Level of education	Contraceptive method use								Number of women
	Any method	Sterilization		IUD	DMPA	Pill	Condom	Withdrawal	
		Female	Male						
Illiterate	69.2	29.2	1.7	4.2	5.6	17.9	2.1	7.6	27,677
Primary	75.4	19.0	3.0	8.3	2.9	20.9	5.0	15.6	29,724
Secondary	75.2	10.0	2.9	11.0	1.6	19.7	7.3	21.9	16,170
Diploma or higher	74.6	6.6	3.1	11.2	0.6	14.1	10.5	27.2	13,099

of fertility. The balance between male and female sterilization is higher at the lower parities (Table 6.7).

Using hormonal methods including the pill and DMPA is high among women with one to three children and then decreases among those who have had four and more. The peak of prevalence for the IUD is found among women with two children and then among those who have had only one child. These patterns are consistent with these methods being used for the widespread spacing of births as described in Chapter 4.

The usage of condoms and withdrawal according to the number of children born is similar to that of the hormonal methods and the IUD. Thus these methods also seem to be used for spacing. However, these methods, particularly withdrawal, are also used before the birth of the first child by a minority of women. As observed in Chapter 4, delay of the first birth within marriage is an emerging feature of Iranian fertility particularly in Tehran City.

Education Level of Women

Variation in the use of any method of contraception was small across the various levels of education (Table 6.8). Use was a little less common for illiterate women than for others but this may have been due to their residence in provinces such as Sistan & Baluchistan that had lower levels of usage.

Of more interest are the differences by education in the type of method used. As education level rises, women are much more likely to use withdrawal or condoms and much less likely to use the modern methods delivered by the government's family planning program. The use of female sterilization (but not male sterilization) falls sharply as the education levels rises.

This result may mean that women who are illiterate have more children and turn to sterilization to stop childbearing. The second point is that educated women may be more knowledgeable about the side effects of hormonal methods and they may prefer to use a traditional method that has no physiological impact, and in which they are supported by their husbands. There is also a strong hypothesis that abortion is used as a backup to withdrawal by better-off women in urban areas who in turn have better access to abortion providers. Finally, educated women may be less inclined to make use of the government-delivered program and more use of private services.

Reasons for Not Using Contraception

At the national level, around 26% of currently married women aged 15–49 were not using any method of contraception at the time of the IDHS in 2000. Only 6% of them were pregnant; the remaining 20% were not using for other reasons. Reasons for not using contraception can be categorised into three main groups as shown in Table 6.9.

1. Fertility-related reasons include two sub-groups: first, not being physiologically exposed to the risk of pregnancy because of infecundity caused by hysterectomy or menopause, primary infertility, secondary infertility, or because of infrequent or no sexual relationship, or being in a state of post-partum sexual abstinence or lactation amenorrhea; second, being pregnant or trying to become pregnant

Table 6.9 Percentage of currently married women 15–49 not using contraception by demographic characteristics, Iran, 2000 (The 2000 Iran Demographic and Health Survey)

	Age group			
Reason for non-use	15–24	25–34	35–49	Total
Hysterectomy and menopause	0.0	0.5	30.5	9.5
Primary infertility	5.6	9.1	7.6	7.2
Secondary infertility	1.3	7.7	18.3	8.3
No or irregular sexual relationship	31.2	12.3	11.7	19.3
Postpartum abstinence, breastfeeding and amenorrhea	7.4	11.8	3.0	7.6
Currently pregnant (intended) or wanted to get pregnant	41.6	35.5	6.6	29.2
Currently pregnant (unintended)	6.5	11.4	3.6	7.2
Health concerns, fear of side effect, illness, inconvenient use of particular method	2.0	6.8	9.6	5.7
Opposition, lack of knowledge, lack of accessibility due to cost or distance, other and unspecified	4.4	5.0	9.1	6.0
Total	100	100	100	100

2. Contraceptive method-related reasons include health concerns, side effects and fear of side effects, and difficulty in using a specific method.
3. Personal reasons include opposition by a woman, her husband or his family to family planning. This category also includes those women not using contraception due to lack of knowledge about using contraception as well as lack of knowledge about how to access family planning services. Another reason included in this category is inaccessibility of the method or service provider due to cost or distance. A very small percentage of the respondents could not explain why they were not using contraception and these women are also included in this category.

It should be reiterated that, in Iran, free family planning is available within 1 hour walk for around 90% of people. Mobile providers (public sector) service remote locations. Cost is rarely an access issue except for women who want specific methods, such as Norplant or a specific brand of the pill not available through the government's family planning service but available only through the private sector.

As expected, the reasons for not using contraception vary substantially by the age of the woman. For older women, non-users are concentrated in the categories of hysterectomy, menopause, primary and secondary infertility and no or irregular sexual relationship. These reasons accounted for 68% of non-use of contraception among women aged 35–49. In the middle age range, 25–34, the reasons for non-use are dominated by pregnancy related reasons such as being pregnant, wanting to become pregnant or postpartum abstinence, breastfeeding and amenorrhea. These account for 59% of all reasons for non-use in this age group.

For those aged 15–24, pregnancy related reasons were also the most important (56% of non-use), but having no sexual relationship or an irregular sexual relationship was also surprisingly high at 31% of non-users and 14% of all married women aged 15–24. This may have been because their husbands were in military service at the time. All Iranian men from age 19 are required to undertake 22 months of military service. This service can be delayed while education is in progress but marriage is not a reason for exemption. Also, in some Iranian cultures, it is not unusual for the (usually very young) wife to remain with her parents in the first years of marriage and not live with her husband. Such couples may not have begun their sexual relationship or have a very irregular relationship. Finally, some women or their husbands may be studying at a university that is far away from the couple's place of residence or the husband may be working in a distant place.

Determinants of Contraceptive Use

Bivariate analyses of contraceptive use revealed that women with different social and demographic characteristics have different contraceptive use patterns, but correlations between the explanatory variables obscure the interpretation of observed bivariate relationships. What is required is multivariate analysis to explore the impact of each factor when other determinants are taken into account. Logistic regression and multinomial regression are next used to determine whether the associations between contraceptive use and women's characteristics are independent of the impact of other demographic characteristics of women. Logistic regression is used to assess the likelihood of using any type of contraception in association with different demographic characteristics, and the odds ratio of using modern contraception versus traditional methods in association with women's characteristics. The odds ratios are statistically tested in the presence of various factors that show the probability of the measure within a 95% confidence interval. Multinomial logistic regression is applied to examine the full patterns of contraceptive use simultaneously, for example, the likelihood of non-contraceptive use, temporary modern contraceptive use, traditional method use, and permanent or sterilization use. The result of the odds ratio in multinomial logistic regression can be better interpreted by applying multiple classification analysis (MCA) that provides a clearer graphic representation of the differences (Retherford and Choe 1993).

Contraceptive Users Versus Non-Users, Traditional Versus Modern

Table 6.10 shows the likelihood of using any type of contraception compared to non-use of contraception, and also the likelihood of using a modern contraceptive versus traditional methods. Using logistic regression, controlling for the number of children, level of education and place of residence, women aged 25–34 were 24% more likely than married women aged 15–24 to use contraception. Older women (35–49) were 25% less likely than those aged 15–24 to be using a contraceptive method to avoid pregnancy. When modern contraceptive users are examined versus traditional users, both women in the middle and older age groups were less likely to use modern contraception than women in the age group 15–24.

A relation between contraceptive practice and number of children remains after controlling for other variables. About 90% of Iranian couples perceive ideal fertility to be represented by two children, and consider four children to be a large family (Abbasi-Shavazi et al. 2004). Women with three children are 17% more likely to use any method of contraception than women who have two children. The efficacy of methods used is also higher for those with three children; women with three children are 40% more likely to use modern than traditional methods than women with two children. The likelihood of using any form of modern contraception versus traditional methods among women with more than three children is considerably higher than for women in other categories. Women who have four or more children are 2.7 times more likely to use a modern contraceptive than a traditional method compared to the reference category of women who have two children. Those with no children or one child had a low usage of contraction compared to those with two

Table 6.10 Odds ratios indicating the likelihood of current use of any form of contraception among currently married women 15–49, and using a modern method among contraceptive users by selected factors (The 2000 Iran Demographic and Health Survey)

Variables in the equation		Any method users vs non-users		Modern method users vs traditional users	
Age group	15–24 (Ref.)				
	25–34	**	1.24	**	0.81
	35–49	**	0.75	**	0.47
Number of Children	0–1	**	0.16	**	0.65
	2 (ref.)				
	3	**	1.17	**	1.40
	4+	**	1.61	**	2.70
Level of Education	Illiterate (Ref.)				
	Primary	**	2.14	**	0.58
	Secondary	**	2.95	**	
	Diploma or university	**	3.49	**	0.40
Area of Residence	Rural (ref.)				
	Urban	**	1.38	**	0.65
Region	Gilan and Tehran City, TFR < 1.5 (ref.)				
	Provinces with TFR = 1.7–2.1		1.00	**	1.74
	Provinces with TFR = 2.2–2.4	**	0.66	**	1.59
	Provinces with TFR = 2.5–2.7	**	0.62	**	1.34
	Sistan and Baluchistan TFR = 4.1	**	0.20	**	2.30
	Constant	**	3.01	**	6.32
Cases included in Analysis		82,317		62,275	

* Significant at level $0.01 < P \leq 0.05$.
** Significant at level $P \leq 0.01$.

children and, if they were using a method, it was much more likely to be a traditional method.

Table 6.8 indicated only a very small impact of education level upon contraceptive usage. However, after controlling for place of residence, age, and number of children, education level has a very strong impact upon whether a woman is using contraception or not. Usage rises strongly as the education level rises. Interestingly, there is a negative relationship between the likelihood of using modern methods and increasing levels of education. Among contraceptive users, women with primary education are 40% less likely than illiterate women to practise a modern contraceptive method (as opposed to a traditional form), and the likelihood of using a modern method decreases by about 52–60% for women with tertiary education.

The likelihood of using modern rather than traditional methods is higher in rural areas than in urban areas, but women living in urban areas are 38% more likely to use any form of contraception to avoid pregnancy.

In the logistic regression model, provinces were divided into five categories to examine contraceptive use differentials according to the provincial level of fertility. Gilan and Tehran City are considered as the reference category having the lowest fertility in the country. After controlling for age, education, rural/urban residence and the number of children, there is no difference in overall usage between provinces that have near-replacement fertility (TFR = 1.7–2.1) and Gilan and Tehran City. However, users in the near-replacement fertility provinces are 74% more likely to use a modern than a traditional method than women in Gilan and Tehran City. As the fertility level rises in a province, the likelihood of practising contraception falls but the level of usage of modern contraception among users remains higher than in Gilan and Tehran City.

The results confirm that use of traditional methods is more prevalent in the provinces with the lowest levels of fertility.

Conclusion

Use of modern contraception had increased to 26% by 1976, remained stable during the 1980s (27% in 1989), but after the revival of the family planning program, increased sharply to 56% in 2000. Taking the traditional methods into account, around 74% of married women in Iran were using any method of contraception in 2000. The sharp rise in the use of contraception in the late 1980s and during the 1990s indicates the high demand for contraception to control fertility. In 1989, the Iranian Government committed to provide comprehensive family planning services that were free of charge. The level of contraceptive use has levelled off since the mid 1990s but at a level that approaches the highest possible level of contraceptive for the country as a whole. Around 6% of non-users were pregnant and around 10% were infecund or had experienced sub-infecundity and did not need to use contraception to control their fertility. Only 4% of women desired to become pregnant. Only a small proportion of women (around 5%) had an unmet need for contraception.

The analysis of method mix confirmed that the pill has been the most commonly used method followed by female sterilization and traditional methods. However, the proportion of those who were using the pill and traditional methods has declined slightly since the mid 1990s while the use of long-term methods such as female and male sterilization, IUD, and DMPA has risen over time. One of the reasons for this trend may be that women have met their desired number of children at relatively young ages and have been more willing to use long-term methods of contraception in recent years.

Traditional methods (overwhelmingly withdrawal) are the second most commonly used method of contraception at 22% of currently married women. Usage of traditional methods was higher for those with higher levels of education and for those living in urban areas. Of particular note is the high prevalence of traditional methods in the low fertility provinces, 30% in Tehran City and 24% in Gilan. This situation is similar to Italy where there is a high level of usage of traditional methods while the fertility is at very low levels (Dalla Zuanna et al. 2005). One of the reasons for this association is that couples are more educated and have more knowledge of contraceptive use. It may also be possible that traditional methods are used in combination with other methods of contraception or abortion as a result of which fertility has declined to a low level. The use of traditional methods probably has a long history among higher educated, urban women. The proportion of women using traditional methods was not affected by the introduction of the family planning program in 1989 even though the program was focussed on the delivery of modern methods. It may be that withdrawal is an established part of the sexuality of couples in this sub-group. More qualitative research is needed to shed light on this issue.

As expected, age was an important factor determining the use of contraception, but this was mainly due to the number of children as older women were more likely to use longer-term methods or sterilization. The number of children clearly explained the type of method used. The use of any type of hormonal method or IUD among women with no children was low. This may have been due to a perceived fear of the risk of infecundity. The use of sterilization also confirmed the patterns of parity progression ratios discussed in Chapter 4 as a high proportion of women with three children had undergone sterilization to stop their childbearing. Education was also an important factor affecting the level and pattern of contraceptive use. While the use of any type of birth-control method increased with the level of education, the use of modern methods was less prevalent among those with higher levels of education. This is particularly the case for use of hormonal methods among women with tertiary education. This could be due to their perceptions of side effects of these methods. These women are able to acquire information from various sources about the side effects of the methods and then choose the best method for themselves. This helps to explain why the use of traditional methods was higher among the highly educated.

There was variation in contraceptive use by place of residence, ethnicity and religion. When ethnicity and religion were considered in different contexts, the levels and patterns of contraceptive use differed, suggesting that the level of development has an impact on the contraceptive behaviour of women, although the varying cultures of ethnic and religious groups are likely also to have played a role. The levels, trends and patterns of contraceptive use in Iran and the low fertility provinces were examined in this chapter. Using the 2000 IDHS, Erfani and McQuillan (2008: 459) found that contraception has the largest effect on fertility, accounting for 61 percent of the reduction in fertility from its theoretical maximum. However, a central question is how and under what conditions women have used contraception to delay the initiation of childbearing and/or to space their births, and finally what methods were used to stop childbearing. This will be examined in the following chapter.

References

Abbasi-Shavazi MJ, Khademzadeh A (2004) Determinants of withdrawal use in Rasht city: a qualitative study (Persian). J Fertil Infertil 5(4):323–337

Abbasi-Shavazi MJ, Hosseini-Chavoshi M, McDonald PF, Delavar B (2004) Fertility transition in Iran: evidence from four selected provinces (Persian). Iran Ministry of Health and Medical Education, Tehran

Agha H (1985) Study of fertility in Iran and its relation with socio-economic indicators based on the Iran Fertility Survey (Persian). Population Studies Center, University of Shiraz, Shiraz

Aghajanian A (1994) Family planning and contraceptive use in Iran, 1967–1992. Int Fam Plann Perspect 20(2):66–69

Aghajanian A, Mehryar A (1999) Fertility, contraceptive use and family planning program activity in the Islamic Republic of Iran: 1976–1996. Int Fam Plann Perspect 25(2):98–102
Balaiah D, Naik DD, Ghule M, Tapase P (2005) Determinants of spacing contraceptive use among couples in Mumbai: a male perspective. J Biosoc Sci 37(6):689–704
Dalla Zuanna G, de Rose A, Racioppi F (2005) Low fertility and limited diffusion of modern contraception in Italy during the second half of the twentieth century. J Popul Res 22(1):21–48
Degraff DS, Bilsborrow RE, Guilkey DK (1997) Community-level determinants of contraceptive use in the Philippines: a structural analysis. Demography 34(3):385–398
Erfani A, McQuillan K (2008) Rapid fertility decline in Iran: Analysis of intermediate variables, Journal of Biosocial Sciences 40(3):459–478
Gribble JN (2003) The standard days method of family planning: a response to Cairo. Int Fam Plann Perspect 29(4):188–191
Hosseini-Chavoshi M (2007) Fertility regulation in Iran: An analysis of trends, levels and correlates. Ph.D. thesis in Demography, Australian Demographic and Social Research Institute, The Australian National University, Canberra
Hosseini-Chavoshi M, Abbasi-Shavazi MJ, McDonald PF (2004) Women's autonomy and reproductive behaviour in Iran. In: 12th Biennial Conference of the Australian Population Association: Population and Society: Issues, Research, Policy, The Australian National University, Canberra
Karra MV, Stark NN, Wolf J (1997) Male involvement in family planning: a case study spanning five generations of a South Indian family. Stud Fam Plann 28(1):24–34
Koc I (2000) Determinants of contraceptive use and method choice in Turkey. J Biosoc Sci 32(3):329–342
Lavecchia C, Decarli A, Parazzini F, Gentile A, Negri E, Franceschi S (1986) Determinants of oral-contraceptive use in Northern Italy. Contraception 34(2):145–156
Lutalo T, Kidugavu M, Wawer MJ, Serwadda D, Zabin LS, Gray RH (2000) Trends and determinants of contraceptive use in Rakai District, Uganda, 1995–98. Stud Fam Plann 31(3):217–227
Mahmud M, Islam MM (1995) Adolescent contraceptive use and its determinants in Bangladesh – evidence from Bangladesh fertility survey 1989. Contraception 52(3):181–186
Malekafzali H (1992) Knowledge, attitude and practice of urban married women 15–49 years old in family planning. J Health 3:1–3
Mehryar A (2005) Shi'ite teachings, pragmatism and fertility change in Iran. In: Jones G, Karim M (eds) Islam, the state and population. Hurst, London, pp 118–156
Ministry of Health (1990) Knowledge, attitude and practice survey: situation analysis on reproductive and family planning behaviour among Iranian women aged 15–45. Unpublished report existing in the Archive of Family Health Department. Iran Ministry of Health, Tehran
Ministry of Health (2002) Population and health in the Islamic Republic of Iran (Iran Demographic and Health Survey): October 2000. Iran Ministry of Health, Tehran
Ministry of Health (2003) Country report of the population and family planning program in the Islamic Republic of Iran. Iran Ministry of Health, Tehran
Mosher WD, Bachrach CA (1986) 1st Premarital contraceptive use in the United-States – determinants and trends, 1960–1982. Stud Fam Plann 18(2):83–95
Nortman DL, Hofstatter E (1978) Population and family planning programs: ninth edition. Population Council, New York
Oddens BJ, Lehert P (1997) Determinants of contraceptive use among women of reproductive age in Great Britain and Germany. 1. Demographic factors. J Biosoc Sci 29(4):415–435
Omran AR (1992) Family planning in the legacy of Islam. United Nations Population Fund, Routledge, New York
Retherford RD, Choe MK (1993) Statistical models for causal analysis. Wiley, New York
Ringheim K (1997) Determinants of contraceptive use. National population-based studies in various west European countries – Oddens, BJ. Patient Educ Couns 31(1):91–93
Svare EI, Kjaer SK, Poll P, Bock JE (1997) Determinants for contraceptive use in young, single, Danish women from the general population. Contraception 55(5):287–294
Tuladhar JM (1985) Determinants of contraceptive use in Nepal. J Biosoc Sci 17(2):185–193
Varena C, Crognier E, Bley D, Boetsch G, Baudot P, Baali A, Hilali MK (1996) Determinants of contraceptive use in Morocco: stopping behaviour in traditional populations. J Biosoc Sci 28(1):1–13

Chapter 7
Contraceptive Use Dynamics: Life Time Use*

Introduction

For the first time in Iran, the 2005 Iran Low Fertility Survey collected information on the full history of women's contraceptive use, that is, for every month of their life from the time that they married. These data provide important insights into the changing contraceptive behaviour of successive generations of Iranian married women. The chapter provides a parallel to Chapter 4 that examined the birth histories of women across their lifetimes. The chapter addresses such questions as what contraceptive methods were used by successive generations to stop their childbearing after they had achieved the number of children that they wanted to have, what methods were used to achieve the remarkably long intervals between the first and the second birth and what methods are being used in the emergence of a delay of the first birth within marriage. The chapter also examines to what extent factors such as place of residence, parity or level of education explain the choice of a specific method and the duration of its use at each stage of the reproductive life course.

Data and Methodology

The data analysed in this chapter is from the 2005 ILFS. The quality and sample size of this data set was described in the previous chapter. Eligible respondents in the survey who were defined as ever married women of age 15–54 at the time of the survey were questioned about their pregnancy history and all episodes of contraceptive use since their first marriage. A total of 5,526 women were successfully interviewed in the selected regions that included Gilan, Isfahan and Yazd provinces and the city of Tehran. Data on pregnancy history and contraceptive practice were obtained from a chart recording pregnancy history and its detailed outcomes, and episodes of contraceptive practice and the reasons for stopping each episode,

---

* This chapter is drawn from Hosseini-Chavoshi (2007).

covering the years preceding the survey since first marriage for each woman. This approach allows collection of contraceptive use across the reproductive lives of the sampled women. Starting with the date of first marriage and working forward through time until the time of the interview, the respondents were asked about children ever born, occurrences of any stillbirths, miscarriages or induced abortions, as well as the length of post-partum sexual abstinence, and the duration of breastfeeding. The data set for the analysis was created as follows. Pregnancies based on the recorded pregnancies in the chart were transferred in order to a table including the date of ending pregnancy and its detailed outcome. Then the dates of gestation for each pregnancy were estimated according to the outcome of pregnancy and the woman's estimate of the duration of the pregnancy. For each episode of contraceptive use during the reproductive life time, the respondent was asked: when she had started using the method; how long she had used it; and whether a conception had occurred while she or her husband was using that method; if not, what was the main reason for stopping the method. The duration of post-partum amenorrhoea for each pregnancy was also recorded.

The data from the pregnancy history and the contraceptive history were integrated with attention being given to the time each reproductive event occurred throughout the life of the woman since her first marriage. The data were then processed into monthly records showing the status of the woman at each given month of her marital reproductive life course. Each record represents a month of a woman's life since her marriage and carries demographic information of the woman plus a variable showing reproductive status of the woman in any given month. This status includes one of the three states: whether she was using a form of contraception and, if so, which method; whether she was in a state of pregnancy; or whether she was neither pregnant nor using contraception.

The data in this monthly format are used in this chapter to explore lifetime contraceptive use among women and its association with demographic characteristics of women such as parity and age. Given that the 2005 ILFS was conducted during April and May 2005, information for the year 2005 was excluded. The earliest recorded year of marriage for respondents in the survey was 1960. The Lexis chart shown in Fig. 7.1 illustrates the duration that each marriage cohort presents in the life history data for lifetime contraceptive use. For example, the marriage cohort 1980–1984 is present in the life history data between 20 and 25 years, and complete lifetime contraceptive use can be explored for all women in this cohort for up to 20 years.

The situation of women in terms of fertility control is investigated during the first 5 years (0–4 years), the second 5 years (5–9), the third 5 years (10–14), the fourth 5 years (15–19) and the fifth 5 years period (20–24) of their reproductive life course since their first marriage. The results for these sequential 5-year periods included those women who had experienced at least 60, 120, 180, 240 and 300 months respectively since their first marriage. Thus, the analysis for all 5-year periods up to 25 years was only possible for marriage cohorts before 1980; or the least experience is available for women married in the period 1995–1999, whose lifetime contraceptive use was only investigated for the first 5 years after marriage.

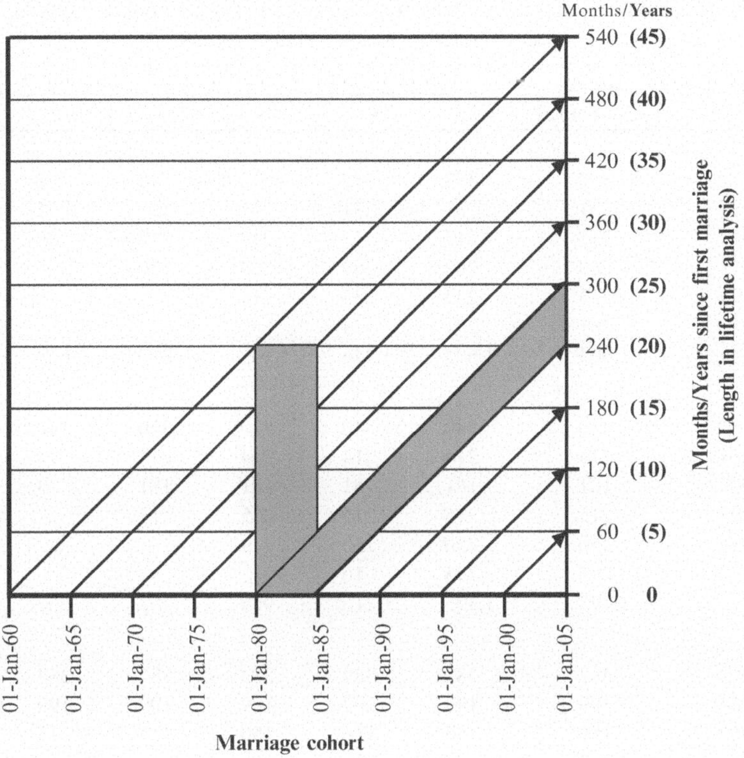

Fig. 7.1 Lexis chart illustrating period and cohort approaches to calculating the lifetime contraceptive use for marriage cohort 1980–1984

Table 7.1 shows the numbers of women eligible for lifetime contraceptive use calculation for each 5-year period after marriage. As the survey was conducted during April and May 2005, only women who married in the first 3 months of the first year of each cohort can be included in the calculation for the first 5 years after marriage. This is indicated by the shaded cells in Table 7.1. These low numbers in each marriage cohort have been excluded from the calculation. In other words, where the marriage cohort is not fully exposed, these cells are excluded.

Lifetime Contraceptive Use

The results from monthly data detailed in Fig. 7.2 show that women in the marriage cohorts of the first and second half of the 1980s were more likely than later cohorts not to be using a contraceptive while they were not pregnant, as well as to be in a pregnant state. This means that the motivation for a child in this period was significantly higher than for later marriage cohorts. In contrast, women who

Table 7.1 Number of women in the 2005 ILFS sample eligible for lifetime contraceptive use calculations in each 5 years after marriage by region and marriage cohort

Region/marriage cohort	Number of women	Years since marriage (eligible each 5 years after marriage)					
		<5	5+	10+	15+	20+	25+
Gilan							
<1980	372	372	372	372	372	372	372
1980–1984	231	231	231	231	231	231	18
1985–1989	217	217	217	217	217	20	
1990–1994	269	269	269	269	20		
1995–1999	233	233	233	14			
2000+	281	281	24				
Total	1,603	1,603	1,346	1,103	840	623	390
Isfahan							
<1980	340	340	340	340	340	340	340
1980–1984	214	214	214	214	214	214	19
1985–1989	181	181	181	181	181	13	
1990–1994	215	215	215	215	17		
1995–1999	250	250	250	19			
2000+	295	295	16				
Total	1,495	1,495	1,216	969	752	567	359
Yazd							
<1980	382	382	382	382	382	382	382
1980–1984	199	199	199	199	199	199	14
1985–1989	156	156	156	156	156	15	
1990–1994	220	220	220	220	14		
1995–1999	240	240	240	16			
2000+	309	309	22				
Total	1,506	1,506	1,219	973	751	596	396
Tehran city							
<1980	250	250	250	250	250	250	250
1980–1984	137	137	137	137	137	137	11
1985–1989	113	113	113	113	113	10	
1990–1994	120	120	120	120	9		
1995–1999	136	136	136	10			
2000+	166	166	12				
Total	922	922	768	630	509	397	261
Combined four regions							
<1980	1,344	1,344	1,344	1,344	1,344	1,344	1,344
1980–1984	781	781	781	781	781	781	62
1985–1989	667	667	667	667	667	58	
1990–1994	824	824	824	824	60		
1995–1999	859	859	859	59			
2000+	1,051	1051	74				
Total	5,526	5,526	4,549	3,675	2,852	2,183	1,406

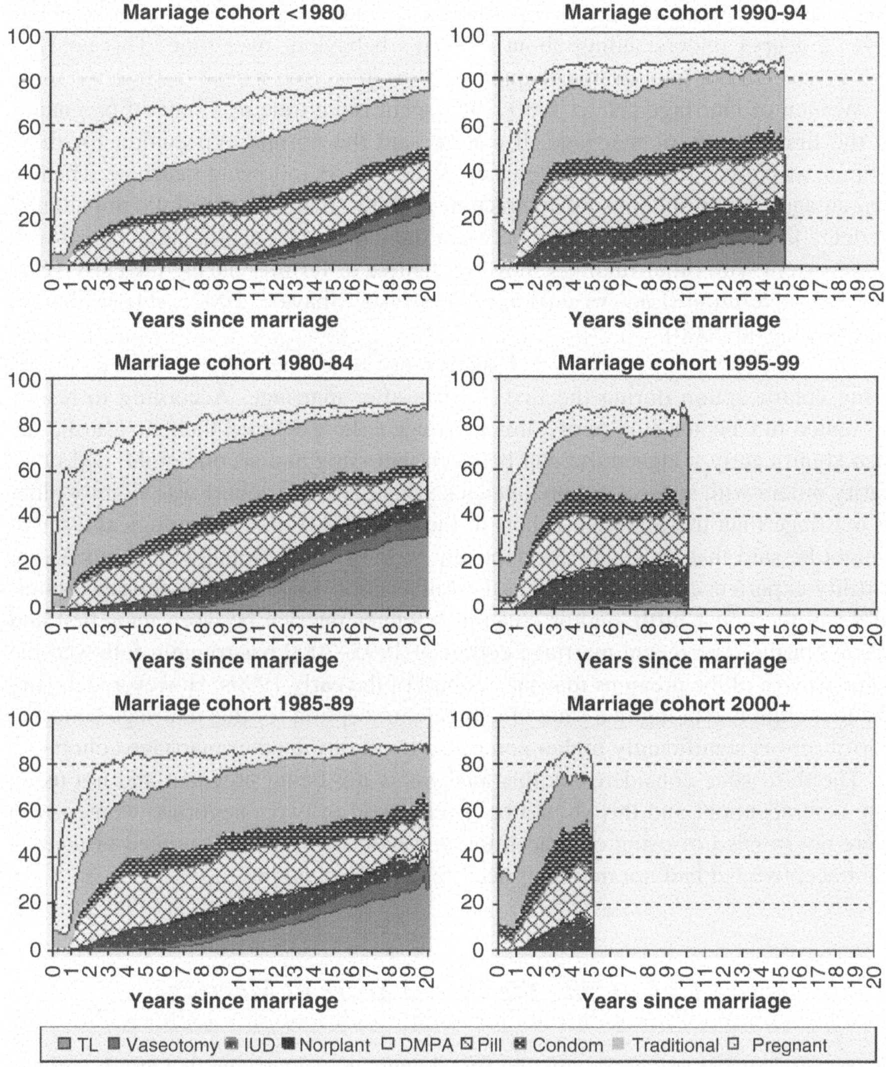

Fig. 7.2 Percentage of each year of marriage using contraception, being pregnant or neither pregnant nor using contraception according to marriage cohort (The 2005 Iran Low Fertility Survey)

married during 1990–1994 were more likely to use a contraceptive and spent most of their first 5 years of reproductive life in protecting themselves against pregnancy. This is true also of the next marriage cohort, 1995–1999, which spent the least time in a state of pregnancy compared to the other marriage cohorts. Exploring the above three categories according to age and parity during the first 5 years after marriage gives a deeper understanding about women's behaviour over time. This analysis will be carried out later in this chapter.

Women of marriage cohort 1980–1984 spent more time in a state of pregnancy in the first 5 years of marriage. It can be said the normal expectation for these women was a first and second pregnancy in the 5 years following marriage. The low percentage of time spent using contraception shows that this cohort did not attempt to delay their first child, or space between their first and second child. This result is consistent with other findings showing the rise of fertility during the early years after the revolution (Ladier-Fouladi 1997; Abbasi-Shavazi, 2002; Abbasi-Shavazi and McDonald 2006).

The marriage cohort 1990–1994 spent more time than other marriage cohorts using contraception during the first 5 years after marriage. According to results presented in Chapter 4 on parity, this marriage cohort delayed their first birth, and also significantly widened the gap between their first and second child, and other parity orders with subsequent pregnancies. This marriage cohort was slightly older at marriage than the marriage cohort in the early 1980s, but in biological terms it cannot be said that they had less exposure to the risk of pregnancy. The different fertility experience is mostly due to the higher motivation of this marriage cohort to delay their first birth, and/or creating a longer interval between their first and second births. The recent marriage cohort of 1995–2000 has roughly followed the same pattern of the previous marriage cohort of the early 1990s. However, delaying the first child and being in a state of using contraception for this marriage cohort at parity zero is significantly higher compared to all of the other marriage cohorts.

The third state considered in this analysis is not being pregnant and not using any contraception, and this should be investigated in two categories: women who were not in need of using contraception and women who were in need of using a contraceptive but had not met their need for family planning.

Contraceptive Use During the First 5 Years of Marriage

In terms of reproductive life, it is the first 5 years after marriage that are the principal childbearing years. Table 7.2 shows that the percentage of months using contraception during the first 5 years following marriage has increased over time. For example, women in the marriage cohorts before 1980 used contraception 24.6% of the time during the first 5 years after marriage and were in a pregnant state for 31% of the first 5 years. This means that during the first 5 years after marriage, women used a form of contraception for a total period of only 15 months, were pregnant for a total period of 19 months and were neither pregnant nor using a contraception for a period of 26 months.

Remarkably, despite a passive family planning program during the 1980s, the time spent using a form of contraception in subsequent marriage cohorts 1980–1984 and 1985–1989 rose to 35% (21 months) and 45.3% (27 months) respectively of the 60-month period. However, the time spent pregnant changed little for the 1980–1984 marriage cohort compared with the previous marriage cohort. Change was considerable for the 1985–1989 cohorts and again for the 1990–1994 cohorts. This supports the observations in Chapters 3 and 4 that fertility had begun to fall at least 5 years before the re-introduction of the family planning program in 1990. In the 1990s, women used a form of contraception for over half of the duration of the first 5 years after their marriage. They were also in a state of pregnancy for only 17–19% of these years. This means that most of these women on average had had one pregnancy.

Contraceptive Use During the Second 5 Years of Marriage

Reproductive behaviour during the second 5 years after marriage (Table 7.3) shows that all marriage cohorts used contraception for longer than they did during the first 5 years following marriage. However, again women who married before 1980 had the shortest duration of using contraception and the longest duration of being in a state of pregnancy. Women who married before 1980 were less likely to be practising contraception in the second 5-year period following marriage, and they were in a state of pregnancy for almost 14 months during that period meaning they had one to two pregnancies during the period. The results among subsequent marriage cohorts vary considerably from the previous cohort. Women who married in the period 1980–1984 practised a form of contraception for 64% of the second 5-year period.

Table 7.2 Percentage distribution of months during first 5 years of marriage using contraception, being pregnant or neither pregnant nor using contraception (The 2005 Iran Low Fertility Survey)

Marriage cohort	Using contraception	Pregnant	Neither pregnant nor using contraception	No. of women
<1980	24.6	31.1	44.3	1,344
1980–1984	35.0	30.0	35.0	781
1985–1989	45.3	24.8	29.9	667
1990–1994	54.1	19.0	26.9	824
1995–1999	55.3	17.0	27.7	859

Table 7.3 Percentage distribution of months during 5–9 years of marriage using contraception, being pregnant or neither pregnant nor using contraception (The 2005 Iran Low Fertility Survey)

Marriage cohort	Using contraception	Pregnant	Neither pregnant nor using contraception	No. of women
<1980	44.5	23.6	31.9	1344
1980–1984	64.2	16.6	19.2	781
1985–1989	73.1	10.5	16.4	667
1990–1994	75.3	10.2	14.5	824

In other words, they used a contraceptive for 38 months out of a 60-month period, and were in a state of pregnancy for almost 10 months in the same period, just over one pregnancy on average. This distribution means that for around 12 months during the same period, these women were not using contraception and were nor pregnant.

Women who married in the period 1985–1994 used contraception for significantly longer, and were pregnant for a significantly shorter duration during the period 5–9 years following marriage. On average, women in this marriage cohort had one or no pregnancy in the second 5-year period. Women or their husbands protected themselves by using a form of contraception to avoid pregnancy for more than 3 years of the second 5-year period after marriage. The widening interval between the first and second birth discussed in Chapter 4 is well explained by the aforementioned result. In Chapter 4, it was concluded that, since 1985, this interval had gradually widened particularly during the 1990s.

Contraceptive Use During the Third 5 Years of Marriage

In Table 7.4, the distribution of months after marriage for the duration of 10–14 years after marriage shows that, as expected, the time spent pregnant has decreased considerably. On average, for those married after 1980, there is less than one pregnancy for each of the 5-year durations in the period 10–14 years after marriage. Women of these cohorts mostly practised contraception during the period 10 or more years after marriage. However, women of the marriage cohorts before 1980 averaged almost two pregnancies during the period 10–14 years after marriage. What is noteworthy here is that women who married during the period 1980–1984 were protecting themselves against pregnancy almost to the same degree as women in the subsequent marriage cohort. This result is important as the marriage of these women coincides with the post-revolution pronatalist ideology by which women were encouraged to have higher fertility. Clearly, they no longer held these motivations in the 1990s.

To conclude, the recent marriage cohorts were more likely to use contraception and less likely to be pregnant or not using contraception. The question that arises is the type of method that these women used during the various stages of their reproductive lifespan to prevent pregnancy. This will be discussed in the following section.

Table 7.4 Percentage distribution of months during 10–14 years of marriage using contraception, being pregnant or neither pregnant nor using contraception (The 2005 Iran Low Fertility Survey)

Marriage cohort	Using contraception	Pregnant	Neither pregnant nor using contraception	No. of women
<1980	56.9	16.7	26.4	1,344
1980–1984	78.6	7.6	13.8	781
1985–1989	81.2	5.3	13.6	667

Lifetime Contraceptive Use: Type of Method

The type of method used during a woman's reproductive life course obviously varies according to the duration of marriage as well as the parity at starting the method. Tables 7.5–7.11 illustrate the type of method used by women during each 5-year period of marriage. In general, as the duration of marriage increases, women are more likely to use contraception for a longer period – obviously due mainly to their increasing parity. Moreover, the percentage of months using contraception in all consecutive 5-year periods after marriage increases over time. For example, the percentage using any form of contraception during the first 5 years of marriage (Table 7.5) increases from 24.6% in the marriage cohort prior to 1980 to 55.3% for the cohort 1985–1990. This trend can also be observed for the next 5-year period after marriage.

Table 7.5 Percentage of months in each 5 years of marriage using any type of contraception (The 2005 Iran Low Fertility Survey)

	Years since first marriage				
Marriage cohort	0–4	5–9	10–14	15–19	20–24
<1980	24.6	44.5	56.9	69.7	75.7
1980–1984	35.0	64.2	78.6	85.3	
1985–1989	45.3	73.1	81.2		
1990–1994	54.1	75.3			
1995–1999	50.3				

Table 7.6 Percentage distribution of months in each 5 years of marriage using a sterilization method (male and female sterilization) (The 2005 Iran Low Fertility Survey)

	Years after marriage				
Marriage cohort	0–4	5–9	10–14	15–19	20–24
<1980	0.0	0.2	4.6	19.0	32.3
1980–1984	0.0	1.7	15.2	33.3	
1985–1989	0.2	4.0	14.1		
1990–1994	0.2	4.2			
1995–1999	0.3				

Table 7.7 Percentage distribution of months in each 5 years of marriage using a modern reversible method (The 2005 Iran Low Fertility Survey)

	Years after marriage				
Marriage cohort	0–4	5–9	10–14	15–19	20–24
<1980	12.9	24.7	27.3	25.5	20.6
1980–1984	18.1	36.4	36.9	27.5	
1985–1989	24.1	41.2	39.0		
1990–1994	30.1	43.1			
1995–1999	33.3				

Table 7.8 Percentage distribution of months in each 5 years of marriage using a hormonal method (pill or DMPA) (The 2005 Iran Low Fertility Survey)

	Years after marriage				
Marriage cohort	0–4	5–9	10–14	15–19	20–24
<1980	8.9	16.9	16.7	15.2	11.4
1980–1984	11.9	21.4	20.7	13.8	
1985–1989	14.9	22.2	20.7		
1990–1994	17.2	22.0			
1995–1999	17.8				

Table 7.9 Percentage distribution of months in each 5 years of marriage using IUD (The 2005 Iran Low Fertility Survey)

	Years after marriage				
Marriage cohort	0–4	5–9	10–14	15–19	20–24
<1980	1.0	2.8	3.9	3.9	3.6
1980–1984	1.8	7.2	9.0	8.1	
1985–1989	4.1	10.4	9.8		
1990–1994	7.6	12.1			
1995–1999	8.2				

Table 7.10 Percentage distribution of months in each 5 years of marriage using condom (The 2005 Iran Low Fertility Survey)

	Years after marriage				
Marriage cohort	0–4	5–9	10–14	15–19	20–24
<1980	2.9	5.0	6.7	6.4	5.6
1980–1984	4.4	7.7	7.2	5.6	
1985–1989	5.2	8.6	8.5		
1990–1994	5.2	9.1			
1995–1999	7.4				

Table 7.11 Percentage distribution of months in each 5 years of marriage using a traditional method (The 2005 Iran Low Fertility Survey)

	Years after marriage				
Marriage cohort	0–4	5–9	10–14	15–19	20–24
<1980	11.8	19.5	24.9	25.1	22.7
1980–1984	16.9	26.1	26.5	24.4	
1985–1989	21.0	27.9	28.1		
1990–1994	23.8	28.0			
1995–1999	21.7				

This means that women's intention to control their fertility is affected by their parity, as well as their motivation to control fertility – which has increased considerably since 1980. Examining the type of method used allows a deeper understanding of how and by which means women have controlled their fertility.

Sterilization Methods

Sterilization methods are almost entirely chosen by couples when they want to limit their childbearing. As a result, it is expected that this method will rarely be chosen during the first 10 years of marriage. Users include only couples that have achieved their ideal number of children during the first years after marriage. The results show that no woman of the marriage cohorts before 1985 used this method during the first 5 years after marriage and only a few women in subsequent marriage cohorts used this method within the first 5 years following marriage. These women may include those with a low ideal fertility, or due to higher age at marriage, women may undergo child bearing immediately following marriage. In the period 5–9 years after marriage, the percentage of months using sterilization methods increased from 0.2% to about 4% across the marriage cohorts. Using a sterilization method is most prevalent after 15 years following marriage (Table 7.6). However, a considerable number of women or their husbands from the marriage cohort 1980–1984 chose to undergo sterilization during the third 5-year period (i.e., 10–14 years).

Marriages that took place in the period 1980–1984 coincided with the first years following the revolutionary government's pronatalist population ideology. This policy encouraged women to have more children and stopped support for family planning. Studies (Ladier-Fouladi 1997; Abbasi-Shavazi and McDonald 2006) have observed the highest level of fertility during this period. Women who married during this period might have been encouraged not to delay childbearing following marriage. The results for sterilization use show that this marriage cohort used sterilization methods a little earlier than the subsequent marriage cohort. For the marriage cohort 1980–1984, sterilization was used for 15.2% of the period 10–14 years after marriage compared with 14.1% for the marriage cohort 1985–1989. The 1980–1984 cohort were encouraged to undergo childbearing earlier in the marriage, but they also stopped childbearing earlier once government policy changed in the 1990s. This result is also supported by the description of the synthetic parity progression results in Chapter 4.

Modern Reversible Contraceptive Methods

Table 7.7 demonstrates that the percentage of months that women have used any form of modern reversible contraception has increased across the marriage cohorts from 12% for those married before 1980 to 33% for those married in the years, 1995–1999. Despite the pronatalism that followed the revolution, the 1980–1984 marriage cohort adopted these methods in the first 5 years of marriage to a greater extent than earlier cohorts and at the relatively high level of 18%. This indicates that a sizeable minority of women were able to obtain these forms of contraception during the pronatalist period and that they were motivated to do so even within the first 5 years of marriage. This supports the view that there was a latent demand for contraception that gradually took on greater meaning during the 1980s as government policy changed.

The longest durations of reversible modern contraception use are observed in the period 5–14 years after marriage. The use declines after 15 years as women make greater use of sterilization methods. Health service providers were instructed that hormonal contraception should not be recommended after 35 years of age (Ministry of Health 1990). Until 1995, the family planning program in the Iranian Ministry of Health followed this viewpoint. After this period, the Ministry of Health no longer promoted age-based limitation for hormonal pill use. Nevertheless, it seems that users continued to move away from hormonal methods at older ages.

Women within 5–14 years after marriage may still be achieving their ideal number of children and opt to use a reversible modern contraceptive to achieve their preferred spacing between children. It is noticeable that women who married between 1985 and 1994 have used a reversible modern contraception for 25–26 months out of the second 5-year period after marriage. This is consistent with the emergence of the very long interval between the first and the second birth. Investigating the type of reversible method that women have used provides valuable insights into how women have changed their preference for reversible methods during their reproductive lives.

Hormonal Methods

The pill is one of the most commonly used reversible forms of contraception among Iranian women and its use is as prevalent as the withdrawal method. Injectable contraception (DMPA) was introduced to the new Iranian family planning program in the early 1990s. While use of DMPA is increasing, the percentage of women using DMPA is less than 5% of women of reproductive age (Ministry of Health 2002). To deal with the low numbers using injectable methods, in this section, pill and injectable methods are combined and these will be discussed as hormonal methods. Hormonal methods are the most common reversible modern contraceptive method used during the reproductive life course of women who married prior to 1980. Except for the first 5-year period after marriage, they used these methods for a total of 8–10 months in each subsequent 5-year period up to 20 years. The use of hormonal methods was a little higher for subsequent marriage cohorts (1980 onwards). However, the levels of usage achieved by the 1980–1984 cohort in the period 5–14 years after marriage were not exceeded by subsequent marriage cohorts (Table 7.8). In the first 5 years after marriage, usage of hormonal methods has gradually increased across time.

IUD

One of the most cost-effective methods of contraception promoted by the Iranian Ministry of Health is the IUD. However, the side effects of IUD use often result in early discontinuation. Moreover, this method has not been recommended by the

Iranian family planning program prior to the first birth. The results show that this method is used for the shortest period compared to other methods during the first 5-year period following marriage. However, using this method has also increased over time. For example, women who married before 1985 used the IUD for less than 2% of the first 5-year period (Table 7.9). This percentage had increased to 8% for marriage cohorts from 1990 onwards. These women are more likely to be those who had at least one child within the first year or two of marriage and then commenced using the IUD for birth spacing.

Using IUD within the second 5-year period after marriage is a little more common and comprises 10–12% of months in the second 5-year period for marriage cohorts after 1984. Like the pill, the IUD was also less commonly used among marriage cohorts prior to 1980 compared to subsequent marriage cohorts. Generally, it can be concluded that over time use of the IUD has increased at a slightly higher rate than for other reversible methods.

Condom

Like the contraceptive pill, the condom was one of the oldest methods introduced by the first family planning program under the Shah's regime. The noticeable result about condom use is that there is a small increase across marriage cohorts in the percentage of months of condom use in each 5-year period following marriage. This method was slightly more prevalent in the first 5-year period after marriage among the cohort 1995–1999 (7.4%) compared to previous cohorts (4–5%). However, condom use in all 5-year periods following marriage is roughly similar among all marriage cohorts (Table 7.10). Overall, condom usage is relatively low.

Traditional Methods

Traditional methods refer almost exclusively to withdrawal. The results (Table 7.11) show that fertility behaviour in relation to use of withdrawal has not changed over time, except for the marriage cohort prior to 1980. Compared to subsequent marriage cohorts, women who married before 1980 made a little less use of traditional methods in the first 10 years of marriage.

The results show that many women rely on withdrawal over their reproductive life course. Its use has always been more common that any other method of contraception in the first 15 years of marriage and is second only to sterilization after 15 years of marriage. Furthermore, practice of this method increased over time among marriage cohorts despite the increasing availability of alternative modern contraception methods. Only for the 1995–1999 cohort in the first 5 years of marriage is there evidence of a small shift from withdrawal to modern reversible methods.

Lifetime Contraceptive Use: Socio-Demographic Influences

Province and the Dynamics of Contraceptive Use

During the period of high fertility prior to 1985, new ideas and methods of fertility control circulated mainly in Tehran. Different levels of knowledge about contraception or aspirations in relation to fertility between women living in different provinces is exemplified in the following interview fragments in the qualitative research associated with this study. A 64 year old woman born and raised in Tehran, and mother of two children explained: “My husband did not want to have more children. He took it upon himself to prevent pregnancy. Sometimes even he asked me to take a douche after our sexual relations”. An Isfahani respondent of similar age and mother of eight children explained: “We had no plan for the number of our children. I did not know at all whether I could prevent pregnancy… we did not think about it at that time”.

Figure 7.3 contrasts the reproductive behaviour of women in each month of the first 12 years of marriage for the four regions included in the Iran Low Fertility Survey. Given the establishment of the new family planning program in 1989 and the extent of fertility decline in the first half of the 1990s, this section splits the time using contraception into two periods: before 1990 and after 1990. Time is split in this way in order to compare the effect of the new family planning program. Comparing the four selected regions indicates that women living in Tehran City demonstrate reproductive behaviour that is different from women living in the other regions both before and after the revival of the official family planning program. However, in all regions, using contraception within 12 years of marriage is considerably higher after 1990 than before 1990. Similarly, in all regions since 1990 women spent less time pregnant than before 1990. Further, the use of sterilization as an indication of early cessation of child bearing is strongly observed since 1990, when free sterilization became available through the family planning program.

In all four provinces, the proportion of time in the first 12 years of marriage spent pregnant or not using a method of contraception falls dramatically for those married after 1990 compared to those married before 1990. Conversely, the usage of any form of contraception expanded significantly in all provinces across the two groupings of years of marriage.

There are striking differences in the contraceptive method used at each duration of marriage in the four regions of the study in spite of the shared characteristic of low fertility. Using contraception within the first 2 years of marriage has been more evident in Tehran City since 1990 than in the other three regions. Forty per cent of those marrying in Tehran City after 1990 began marriage using some form of contraception, mainly withdrawal. Withdrawal was already relatively commonly used in Tehran City in the first 12 years of marriage for those married before 1990 but its use expanded even further after 1990. It was more commonly used than in any other province. The most prevalent modern method used in Tehran City within the 12 years after marriage was the IUD, while the pill was the most prevalent modern contraceptive choice in the other three regions.

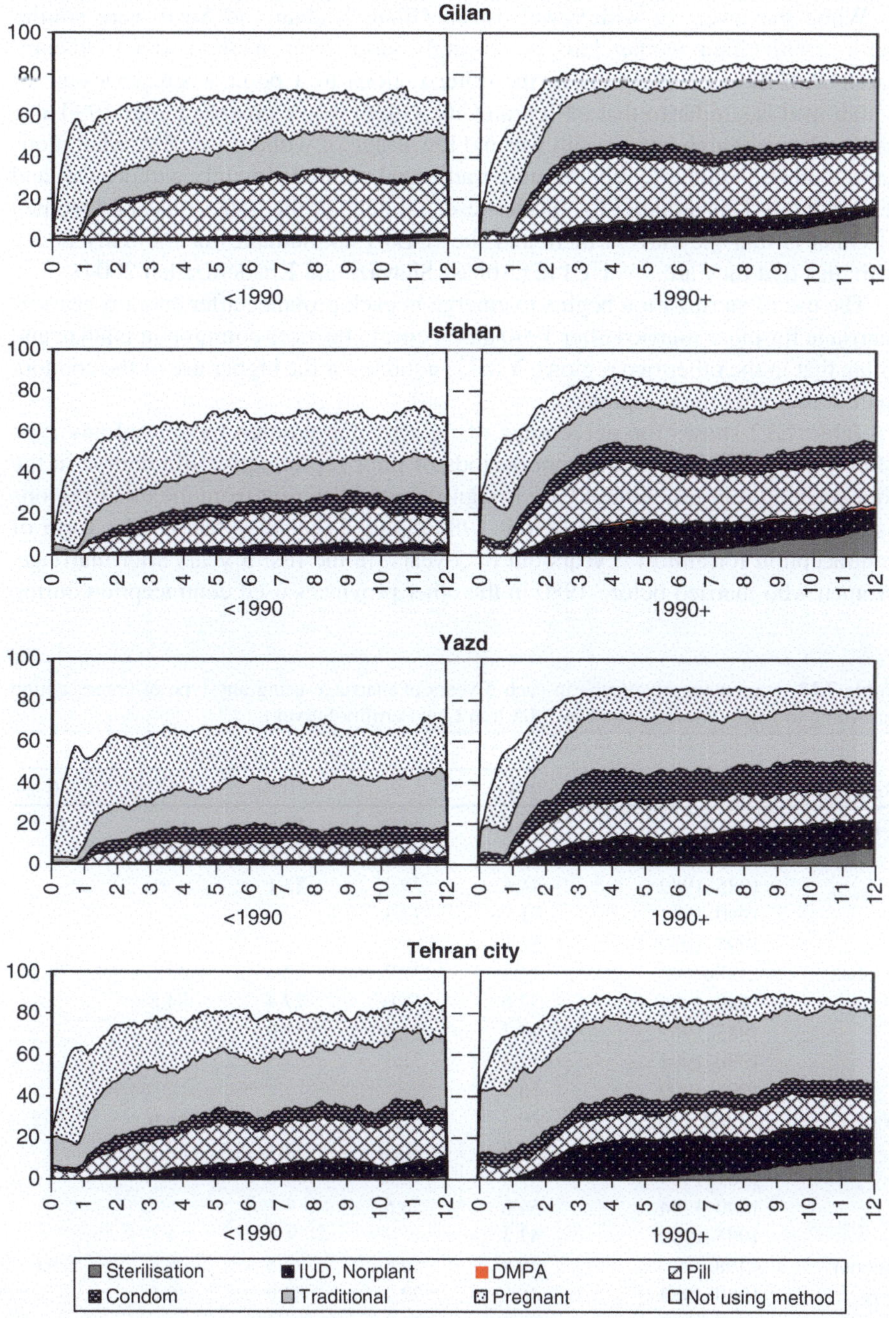

Fig. 7.3 Percentage of each year of marriage spent using contraception, being pregnant or neither pregnant nor using contraception during periods before 1990 and 1990+ by place of residence (The 2005 Iran Low Fertility Survey)

While the levels of withdrawal use in Gilan, Isfahan and Yazd were similar before 1990, Gilani women have increasingly adopted this method after 1990 compared with their counterparts in the other regions to a point where its usage of withdrawal is similar to that of Tehran City. Gilani women married after 1990 also had a relatively high level of pill use and low usage of withdrawal. But, what motivates women in Gilan to rely on more traditional methods (mainly withdrawal) and less on the IUD is a matter for further research. One of the issues raised by women in Gilan is that they are farmers and the IUD is not suitable for the daily heavy activities that they are involved in (Abbasi-Shavazi and Khademzadeh 2004).

The use of sterilization begins to emerge in each province after about 6 years of marriage for those married after 1990 and seems to be more common in Isfahan and Gilan that in the other two regions. Yazd is notable for the higher use of the condom than in the other three regions.

Table 7.12 shows the percentage of months that women have used any type of contraception during different periods of their reproductive life course in the four selected regions. Tehran City is significantly different from the other regions as even women who married before 1980 claimed that they had used a form of contraception for almost 2 years out of 5 years, in the first 5 years after marriage. Women who married before 1980 in the other provinces used contraception during

Table 7.12 Percentage of months in each 5 years of marriage using any type of contraception according to place of residence (The 2005 Iran Low Fertility Survey)

		Years after marriage				
Region	Marriage cohort	0–4	5–9	10–14	15–19	20–24
Gilan	<1980	22.6	45.2	55.6	68.1	71.7
	1980–1984	34.2	62.9	77.1	85.0	
	1985–1989	44.4	73.3	83.1		
	1990–1994	51.5	77.3			
	1995–1999	53.3				
Isfahan	<1980	19.4	39.7	53.6	68.6	78.7
	1980–1984	32.6	64.0	77.4	84.8	
	1985–1989	44.7	71.9	81.9		
	1990–1994	52.3	71.1			
	1995–1999	56.7				
Yazd	<1980	20.7	37.9	50.4	66.0	74.2
	1980–1984	30.7	60.4	77.1	83.4	
	1985–1989	39.3	72.5	77.6		
	1990–1994	54.6	76.6			
	1995–1999	53.3				
Tehran city	<1980	40.8	59.5	72.8	78.4	79.6
	1980–1984	46.3	72.2	84.9	89.2	
	1985–1989	56.3	75.4	81.2		
	1990–1994	62.3	75.7			
	1995–1999	59.8				

the first 5 years of marriage almost half the duration of their counterparts from Tehran City.

For recent cohorts since 1985, women across all four regions demonstrated very similar reproductive behaviour during the second 5 years of marriage: using contraception for almost 42–45 out of the 60 months. Marriage cohorts after 1985 across all regions behave similarly, whereas among marriage cohorts prior to 1985, Tehran was an anomaly with higher usage of contraception. Among Tehran marriage cohorts prior to 1985, women used contraception to prevent pregnancy for 73% of the duration of 10–14 years after marriage, while this percentage for the other three regions was about 50%.

The interesting point about Tehran City is that when these percentages were calculated for the period that women were not in a state of pregnancy, it became clear that Tehrani women married before 1980 practiced contraception significantly more frequently than women in the other three regions in the study – almost 10–20% points higher, while for all women married after 1985, Tehrani contraceptive practice was different only during the first 5 years after marriage.

Among the four studied regions, earlier marriage cohorts in Yazd and Isfahan had almost the same practice of contraception use during the two 5-year periods subsequent to marriage. For example, marriage cohorts before 1980 and 1980–1984 in Yazd and Isfahan provinces have the same durations of contraceptive use in the first 5 years after marriage (about 20% for the cohort prior to 1980, and 30–32% for the cohort 1980–1984). However, among women married after 1985, women from Isfahan and Yazd moved closer to practices in Gilan and Tehran City by practising longer contraception use in each 5-year period following marriage.

For the most recent time period (the last numbers in each column), the levels of contraceptive use are very similar across all four regions. This is interesting because the level of fertility is lower in Tehran City and Gilan than it is in Isfahan and Yazd. It can be hypothesized that women in Gilan and Tehran City have reached below replacement fertility with the additional use of abortion. Abortion is used in these regions as a back up to contraceptive failure where both regions have a high usage of withdrawal.

When the four provinces are examined based on the duration that women had spent pregnant within the first 5 years following marriage (Table 7.13), women in Tehran City have spent less time in a state of pregnancy across all marriage cohorts compared to the other three provinces. However, the most recent marriage cohorts (since 1990) in all regions have spent about the same duration in a state of pregnancy during the first 10 years after marriage. Comparing Gilan and Tehran City with Isfahan and Yazd, women of earlier marriage cohorts in the former two provinces had spent less time in a state of pregnancy in the 10 years following marriage than their counterparts in the latter two provinces. That Tehran City and Gilan have had the lowest fertility in the country is the result of greater levels of fertility control observed among women who married even before 1985.

Table 7.13 Percentage of months in each 5 years of marriage being pregnant (The 2005 Iran Low Fertility Survey)

		Years after marriage				
Region	Marriage cohort	0–4	5–9	10–14	15–19	20–24
Gilan	<1980	31.9	21.7	15.8	7.4	2.2
	1980–1984	31.5	17.0	7.2	2.5	
	1985–1989	26.1	10.6	4.2		
	1990–1994	19.7	7.8			
	1995–1999	17.4				
Isfahan	<1980	30.7	26.0	18.6	9.5	3.4
	1980–1984	28.6	16.4	8.0	3.3	
	1985–1989	24.4	11.2	6.2		
	1990–1994	18.7	10.5			
	1995–1999	16.9				
Yazd	<1980	33.5	26.6	19.3	10.4	4.2
	1980–1984	33.5	19.1	8.7	4.3	
	1985–1989	26.6	11.1	7.2		
	1990–1994	19.7	12.3			
	1995–1999	17.5				
Tehran city	<1980	26.5	18.8	11.7	6.1	1.8
	1980–1984	24.8	12.7	5.7	1.6	
	1985–1989	20.6	8.8	3.3		
	1990–1994	16.8	11.2			
	1995–1999	15.9				

Parity and the Dynamics of Contraceptive Use

The number of children is one of the most important factors influencing women's choice of contraception to space or limit. Figure 7.4 provides a parity-specific view of the use of contraception across the years of marriage for various marriage cohorts. Remaining at parity zero within the first 5 years of marriage rose across the marriage cohorts only from 23 to 28 months, with the increased gap being due to use of contraception among recent marriage cohorts. This means that those at zero parity level are still unlikely to use a contraceptive method. Further, a very small percentage of women had not given birth after 5 years of marriage and there is little sign of contraception use at the level of zero parity within the 5–14 year period following marriage. By this period, a woman is probably sure about her potential fertility, and it is rare that women seek to use a form of contraception after 5 years following marriage if they have not yet given birth.

The most significant change across marriage cohort in the first 5 years of marriage is the increase in the duration of contraception use after the birth of the first child. This duration increases from around 7 months for the pre-1908 marriage cohorts to more than 24 months for the 1995–1999 marriage cohort. Going forward to the second 5 years of marriage, the duration off use of contraception following the first birth is again an important aspect of the changes across cohorts increasing

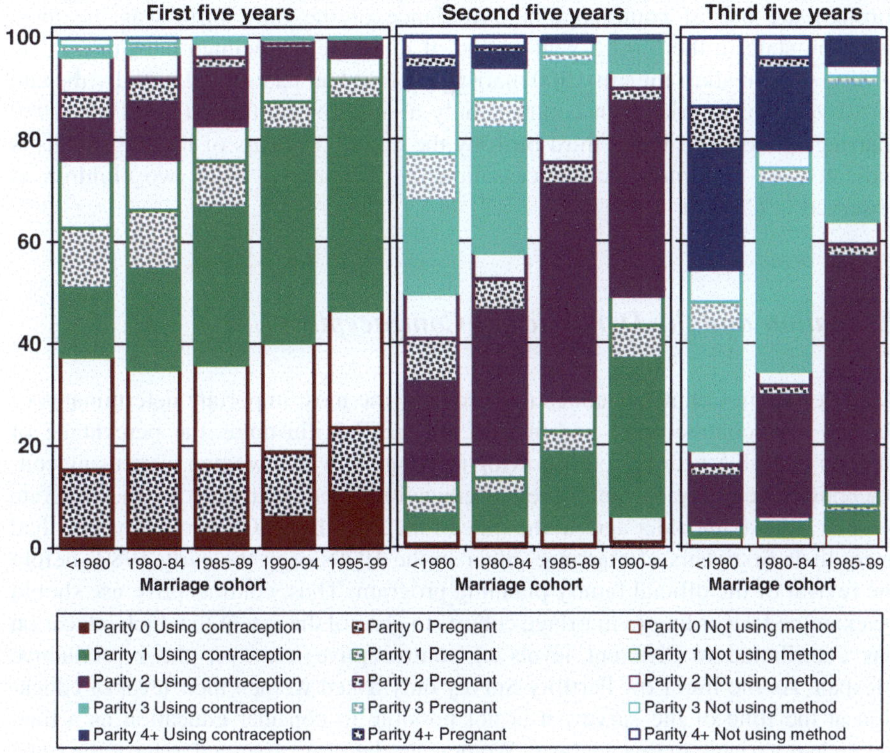

Fig. 7.4 Percentage of months in each 5 years of marriage using contraception by parity at time of using the method according to marriage cohort (The 2005 Iran Low Fertility Survey)

from about 2 months for the pre-1980 marriage cohorts to about 18 months for the 1990–1994 cohort. The pattern of the 1990s can be expressed in terms of women setting out to avoid first pregnancy for a short time, falling pregnant and then commencing a long period of spacing between their first and second children. In total, the 1990–1994 used contraception for about 44 months during the 10-year period following their marriage in order to delay their second child. This pattern is consistent with the emergence of a long interval between the first and second births as discussed in the analysis of parity progression in Chapter 4. Being pregnant with the second child consequently drops away as a state of being for Iranian women in the first 5 years of marriage. Indeed, by the 1990–1994 marriage cohort, Iranian women were twice as likely to have had their second birth in the second 5-year period after marriage than pre-1980 marriage cohorts who were well into having their third births within the first 5 years of marriage.

In the second 5 years of marriage, not only does using contraception after a first birth increase substantially across marriage cohorts, so also does the use of contraception after a second birth. Indeed the 1990–1994 marriage cohort spent most of the second 5 years of marriage either avoiding the second or the third birth through the use of contraception. Avoidance of the third birth was the most common state in the third 5-year period of marriage for women born in the late 1980s. Almost all of the pre-1980 marriage cohort had had a third birth by the end of 10 years of marriage. In contrast, only a small proportion of the 1985–1989 marriage cohort had had a third birth by the end of 15 years of marriage. This is indicative of the emergence of cessation of childbearing after two children as observed in Chapter 4.

Education and the Dynamics of Contraceptive Use

As observed in Chapter 6, education is one of the most important determinants of fertility and contraceptive use in Iran. Figure 7.5 illustrates the percentage of months in each 5-year period following marriage in which women were using contraception according to their level of education. Note that most of the illiterate women were at the older ages at the time of the 2005 ILFS. Consequently, they had spent their first years of marriage either in the 1970s or in the early 1980s before the revival of the official family planning program. Thus, contraceptive use should be examined according to marriage cohorts to control the extent to which education has contributed to different levels of contraceptive use over the reproductive lifespan. As the Iran Low Fertility Survey only asked women their level of education at the time of the survey, it is not possible to consider education as a time dependent variable in this analysis. Women are therefore assumed to have the same level of education in the past as the level recorded at the time of the survey.

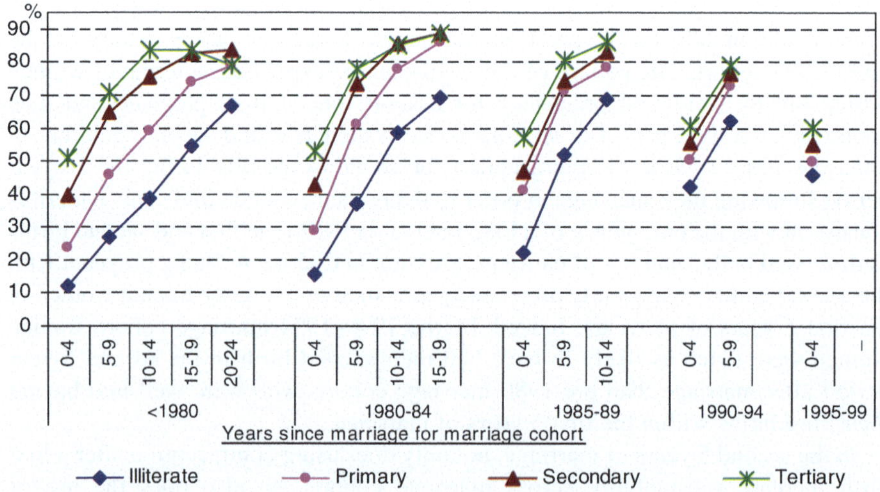

Fig. 7.5 Percentage of months in each 5 years of marriage using contraception according to level of education by marriage cohort (The 2005 Iran Low Fertility Survey)

As depicted in Fig. 7.5, in general, illiterate women were less likely to use contraception at any period of their marital life course as compared with women of other levels of education. The difference in contraceptive uptake is particularly noticeable for the two earlier marriage cohorts: before 1980s and 1980–1984. For instance, illiterate women who married prior to 1980, spent only a small proportion of their first 5 years of marriage (10%) using some form of contraception, while those with primary, secondary, and tertiary levels of education, spent around 25%, 38% and 50% of the first 5 years of marriage using contraception, respectively.

Prior to the revolution, there was a significant difference in contraceptive use between women who were illiterate and those who had a primary and secondary level of education. The gap between those who had secondary education and tertiary education was small. However, for almost all marriage cohorts after the revolution, particularly after 1990, the difference in contraceptive uptake between the levels of education (primary, secondary, and tertiary) reduced considerably. As discussed in Chapter 2, the health network system in Iran was established in the early 1980s and provided access to health education in rural areas where women had lower levels of education.

In brief, contraceptive use has been related to education; the higher the level of education, the more likely the use of contraception. However, the differences by education have become much smaller across marriage cohorts. It should also be noted that the level of education increased after the revolution and the vast majority of younger women are literate and have access to a higher level of education. Only a small proportion of women of recent marriage cohorts are illiterate. The other conclusion to be drawn is that women of all social classes with different levels of education have access to family planning knowledge across the country.

Conclusion and Summary

This chapter investigated the duration of use of contraception by examining the status of a woman at each month of her reproductive life from 1980 onwards. The 2005 ILFS was used for this analysis. The duration of marriage for each woman was divided into months, and for each month, three categories were considered: using a form of contraception, being in a state of pregnancy, and neither pregnant nor using contraception. Moreover, for each month, the type of contraceptive use was also studied. The findings of the chapter can be summarized as follows.

Women in the marriage cohorts of the first and second half of the 1980s were more likely to be pregnant and not using contraception in the first 5 years of marriage, while, women who married during 1990–1994 and 1995–1999 were more likely to use a contraceptive and to spend a considerable time protecting against pregnancy.

The methods of contraception used in each year of marriage differ substantially across the four selected provinces in spite of the shared characteristic of low fertility. Using contraception within the first 2 years of marriage has been of significance mostly in Tehran City since 1990 rather than in the other three regions. The popularity of the IUD in Tehran City within the first 12 years after marriage is higher than in other regions where the pill has been the most popular modern method used during the same period of marriage. Since 1990, women in Gilan increasingly adopted withdrawal in spite of the free availability of modern methods. However, the use of withdrawal was even higher in Tehran City.

The analysis by method showed that women in the later marriage cohorts used sterilization extensively within the third and fourth 5-year period following marriage. However, the percentage of months that women have used any form of modern reversible contraception has increased during each 5-year period of marriage since 1980.

The pill was found to be the most common reversible modern contraceptive method used during the reproductive life course of women who married prior to 1980. The IUD was used least compared to other methods during the first 5-year period following marriage. However, the use of the IUD has increased over time.

While the methods used may vary across provinces, in total, there was convergence across time in the proportions using any method. There was also convergence in usage rates across different levels of education. This indicates the emergence of a pattern in these low fertility provinces whereby women delay the first birth for a short period then delay the second birth for a very long period. Most then have the second birth in the second 5 years of their marriage and then stop childbearing. The long delay of the second birth means that women are older at the second birth than they otherwise would have been. This enables an increasing proportion to adopt sterilization following their second birth.

References

Abbasi-Shavazi MJ (2002) Convergence of fertility behaviours in Iran: provincial fertility levels, trends and patterns in Iran (Persian). Social Sci J 18:201–231

Abbasi-Shavazi MJ, Khademzadeh A (2004) Determinants of withdrawal use in Rasht City: a qualitative study (Persian). J Fertil Infertil 5(4):323–337

Abbasi-Shavazi MJ, McDonald P (2006) The fertility decline in the Islamic Republic of Iran, 1972–2000. Asian Popul Stud 2(3):217–237

Hosseini-Chavoshi M (2007) Fertility regulation in Iran: an analysis of trends, levels and correlates, Ph.D. thesis in Demography, Australian Demographic and Social Research Institute, The Australian National University, Canberra, 2007

Ladier-Fouladi M (1997) The fertility transition in Iran. Popul: Engl Sel 9:191–214

Ministry of Health (1990) Manuals and instructions of the family planning program in Iran (Persian). Ministry of Health, Tehran

Ministry of Health (2002) The Iran's third 5-Year National Health Development Plan: 2000–2004 (Persian). Tehran, Iran Ministry of Health

Chapter 8
A Cohort Perspective on Changes in Family, Fertility Behaviour and Attitudes*

Introduction

Chapters 6 and 7 have shed light on family planning use as the main proximate determinant of fertility. However, given the fact that the onset of fertility decline occurred a few years before the revival of the official family planning program in 1989 and the evidence of use both traditional and modern methods of contraception by a significant minority of women in the years when the official family planning program was dormant, the question arises as to whether other factors such as social change and transformation of attitudes toward family and fertility paved the way for the later success of the family planning program and the phenomenal fertility decline in Iran in recent years. In other words, despite the contribution of the family planning program to an acceleration of the fertility decline during the later 1980s, the program itself can be considered to be a response to the demand for smaller family size observed before the mid-1980s. There is evidence of profound shifts in attitudes toward family-related behaviours in much of the world (Thornton and Freedman 1982; Morgan and Waite 1987) and evidence suggests that changing attitudes toward family life have played a pivotal role in demographic trends (Thornton and Freedman 1982; Thornton 1989; Axinn and Thornton 1993; Thornton and Young-Demarco 2001).

This chapter aims to examine women's reproductive behaviour as well as attitudes toward family and fertility in Iran. The focus of the present chapter will be on four selected provinces of Gilan, Sistan & Baluchistan, West Azarbaijan and Yazd covered in the 2002 Iran Fertility Transition Survey. Among the questions to be addressed are: How do women in contemporary Iran perceive marriage and childbearing? How do these attitudes vary across regions and social groups? Have attitudes of women towards marriage, family and childbearing changed across time? If so, how far have these changes contributed to the fertility decline in Iran? More importantly, if attitudes have changed, how and why did they change? Drawing on

---

* An earlier version of this chapter appeared as the ANU Working Papers in Demography No. 88, and a later version appeared as a book Chapter. See Abbasi-Shavazi et al. (2003), and Abbasi-Shavazi et al. (2008a).

the IFTS data, it is argued here that the Iranian fertility decline has been due to social change at both the macro (societal) and micro (family/individual) levels.

Data and Methodology

The 2002 Iran Fertility Transition Survey (IFTS) is used to document changes in attitudes to family and fertility in four selected provinces.

Social changes can be studied with two distinct forms of period or cohort approaches. Period effects are the result of societal changes influencing all age and cohort groups similarly at one point in time, while marriage and birth cohort effects are defined as the result of social changes that affect only the individuals of one particular birth or marriage cohort (Thornton and Lin 1994:15). There are some difficulties in studying social change using one cross-sectional survey, and particularly compared to having multiple cross-sectional studies. However, with a cross-sectional study, it is possible to categorize people by their year of birth or year of marriage, and then see what their experience was at the same age or life course transition stage. For example, by categorizing people by year of birth, it is possible to see the number of years of education, age at marriage, and work before marriage of the various birth cohorts. Since age is roughly controlled in this case, we can conclude that any differences in education, marriage, work, and attitudes toward childbearing across birth cohorts can be the product of social change.

While the data used in this paper provide many opportunities for the study of family change in Iran, there are some limitations involved as the IFTS covers only married women of childbearing ages. Thornton (1994:419) noted that sample limitations in one cross-sectional study introduce truncation biases of marriage ages across the respective birth and marriage cohorts presented in the study. This is illustrated in Table 8.1.

As can be seen from Table 8.1, the possible ages at marriage of women who were eligible for inclusion in the study vary by birth and marriage cohort. Over time, from the oldest to the youngest, birth cohorts become increasingly limited to women married at younger ages. The marriage cohort truncation problem works

Table 8.1 Ages at marriage that can be represented within different birth and marriage Cohorts in a sample of ever-married women aged 15–49 in 2000

Birth cohort	Possible ages at marriage[a]	Marriage cohort	Possible ages at marriage[a]
1951–55	0–49	1961–65	0–14
1956–60	0–44	1966–70	0–19
1961–65	0–39	1971–75	0–24
1966–70	0–34	1976–80	0–29
1970–75	0–29	1981–85	0–34
1976–80	0–24	1986–90	5–39
1981–85	0–19	1990–95	10–44
		1996–00	15–49

[a] Theoretical marriage ages

in the opposite direction. As marriage cohorts go back in time, the cohorts become increasingly limited to women married at younger ages. If data are tabulated according to both birth and marriage cohorts and birth cohorts are approximately matched to marriage cohorts in calendar time, the range of the results provides some bounds on the magnitudes of the trends observed because the birth cohorts and marriage cohorts are biased (in terms of age at marriage) in opposite directions (Thornton 1994:150). Furthermore, where marriage ages are concentrated in a relatively narrow range and that range is covered by the possible ages at marriage for the birth year or marriage year cohort, then any bias will be small.

As the mean age at marriage has been approximately 20 years, results for marriage cohorts with results for birth cohorts 20 years earlier are compared. The birth and marriage cohorts are defined to represent different periods of social change in Iran.

The different periods of social change in Iran represented by the three time periods (of marriage) are as follows:

Before 1980s: During this period, the first national family planning program was implemented by the Shah, the legal minimum age at marriage for boys and girls was increased, and various programs were implemented to improve the status of women in the society.

1980s: This is the first decade following the Islamic revolution when the country experienced considerable socio-political change. It is also the period of the Iran–Iraq War. The family planning program was suspended, the war situation changed people's lives, a rationing system was introduced to meet people's basic needs, and the legal minimum age at marriage decreased. On the other hand, the egalitarian nature of the revolution led to considerable improvements in education and health systems, and there were major development improvements in rural areas of Iran.

After 1980s: The period from 1990 to the time of the survey in 2002 was more pragmatic in the approach to social and economic issues. The government implemented many infrastructure projects in order to improve the economic situation of the country. The family planning program was revived during this period and the Islamic government supported the family planning program and provided contraceptives to people throughout the country (Abbasi-Shavazi et al. 2002). The election of the Khatami Government in 1997 heralded a democratisation period when various political groups formed and the society experienced profound shifts on political issues. Freedom of speech and expression of different values and attitudes became more prevalent and restrictions on people's personal and individual behaviour became somewhat more limited.

Cohort Fertility in the Four Provinces

In this section, we examine the mean number of children ever born for the various cohorts according to the different periods of social change in Iran (Table 8.2). Comparing the marriage and birth cohorts, there is a close similarity in Gilan for all three periods but, in the other provinces, for the two later time periods when fertility had fallen, the means for the marriage cohorts are significantly lower than the means for the birth cohorts. As Gilan has an older age at marriage than the

Table 8.2 Mean number of children ever born for marriage and birth cohorts by province, 2002 IFTS

Province	Marriage Cohort	Number of women	Mean	Birth Cohort	Number of women	Mean
Gilan	<1980	363	5.1	Before 1960s	366	4.9
	1980s	392	3.2	1960s	451	3.2
	1990+	507	1.5	After 1960s	460	1.6
West Azarbaijan	<1980	389	6.9	Before 1960s	362	6.7
	1980s	429	4.1	1960s	489	4.6
	1990+	496	1.9	After 1960s	517	2.1
Sistan & Baluchistan	<1980	255	7.7	Before 1960s	265	8
	1980s	336	5.5	1960s	433	6.1
	1990+	428	2.3	After 1960s	598	3
Yazd	<1980	428	6.1	Before 1960s	350	6.1
	1980s	376	3.7	1960s	415	4.1
	1990+	435	1.5	After 1960s	484	1.9

other three provinces (see below), this suggests that the 20 year gap used between the marriage and the birth cohorts fits Gilan better than it fits the other provinces. A shorter interval between the birth and marriage cohorts in these three other provinces would have brought the means closer together.

As expected, mean number of children ever born has declined for all cohorts. The very high levels of fertility for the earliest cohort are generally consistent with the cross-sectional estimates of fertility shown in Chapter 3. Across the cohorts, the provincial differences observed across time are also confirmed. The level of fertility of all marriage cohorts in Sistan & Baluchistan was much higher than the levels for other provinces, while marriage cohorts in Gilan have experienced lower fertility than their counterparts in other provinces.

Selected Social and Attitudinal Changes

The following analysis considers cohort trends in selected indicators of social and attitudinal change. This is a preliminary investigation of factors that may have been associated with the fertility decline in Iran. Sought are measures that show strong trends across cohorts that are consistent with the timing of the fall in fertility and are evident in each of the four provinces, albeit with appropriate variation across the provinces. The measures chosen are related to theories of fertility decline and were included in the survey for this reason.

Education

It is very conventional to associate changes in education levels of women with changes in fertility levels. So conventional, in fact, that education plays a part in almost all theoretical approaches to fertility transition. Education is said to provide access to modern ways of thinking, to provide confidence to engage with the modern world, to reduce infant and child mortality, to stimulate higher levels of gender equity within couple relationships and to promote labour force participation of women in the cash economy hence raising the opportunity cost of having children. Education of women may also lead to a greater emphasis on their part on the 'quality' of children as distinct from the quantity of children. Finally, education is a broad indicator of societal modernization. As education levels increase, the educated woman is very likely to be married to an educated man and to be living in an educated society. As already described, the egalitarian nature of the Islamic Revolution led to widespread education of women in Iran especially in rural areas where education for women had been neglected.

Table 8.3 shows the change in education levels of women across birth and marriage cohorts. Based on the analysis of fertility above, we would be looking for a considerable change from cohort to cohort and in every province. This is precisely what the table shows. Education levels change dramatically from one cohort to the next for both marriage and birth cohorts and for all provinces. The change also

Table 8.3 Percentage distribution of birth cohorts by level of education and province, 2002 IFTS

			Level of education				
	Provinces		Illiterate	Primary	Secondary	Diploma and higher	Number of women
Marriage cohort	Gilan	<1980	57.9	24.3	6.5	11.3	363
		1980s	22.8	29.0	28.9	19.3	392
		1990+	5.6	30.8	34.8	28.8	507
	West Azarbaijan	<1980	74.5	16.7	4.8	4.0	389
		1980s	47.7	26.8	18.0	7.5	429
		1990+	23.8	34.8	27.3	14.1	496
	Sistan & Baluchistan	<1980	71.3	17.3	7.3	4.0	255
		1980s	52.0	27.3	12.5	8.2	336
		1990+	42.3	27.0	15.6	15.1	428
	Yazd	<1980	31.3	58.5	3.8	6.4	428
		1980s	13.2	54.2	16.9	15.6	376
		1990+	3.8	34.9	22.8	38.5	435
Birth cohorts	Gilan	<1980	55.6	22.0	6.2	16.3	366
		1980s	22.9	31.4	25.7	20.0	451
		1990+	6.6	30.7	38.2	24.4	460
	West Azarbaijan	<1980	76.5	14.2	3.2	6.2	362
		1980s	50.2	26.8	15.9	7.1	489
		1990+	26.2	34.3	27.6	12.0	517
	Sistan & Baluchistan	<1980	78.4	15.4	1.7	4.5	265
		1980s	60.0	19.0	12.1	8.8	433
		1990+	50.7	27.6	12.7	9.0	598
	Yazd	<1980	34.9	51.9	2.8	10.4	350
		1980s	13.4	59.4	12.4	14.7	415
		1990+	5.4	37.7	24.6	32.3	484

extends across the education distribution. It is not simply a shift from illiteracy to primary education; there are also large shifts at the highest education levels as well.

Differences in education levels between provinces match the fertility differences with the exception that the relatively high education level of women in Yazd, especially in the earliest cohort is not matched by lower fertility. As indicated below, Yazd has family–religious values that may have counter-balanced the effects of its higher education levels. As the above tables show a fairly close relationship between the results for birth cohorts and the results for marriage cohorts, the remainder of the analysis will be based only on marriage cohorts (For comparison of some of the results by birth and marriage cohorts see Abbasi-Shavazi et al. 2003).

Attitudes to Age at Marriage

Respondents in IFTS were asked their views about the lowest age at marriage and the highest age at marriage that would be appropriate for women and for men in their society. The results are shown in Table 8.4. Here, the attitude is a current (2002) attitude and it is evident that there is not much variation across cohorts. From the perspective of theory, we might expect that younger women, particularly given the trends in education, would favour later ages at marriage than older women. If their preferences carried weight, then fertility may fall because of later age at marriage. A preference for later age at marriage might also indicate the perceived availability of alternatives to marriage in the short to medium term, in particular, paid employment.

Only small rises in preferred ages at marriage are apparent across cohorts. This can be interpreted to mean either that attitudes have not changed across time or that they have changed cross-sectionally for all cohorts. At least, the data show

Table 8.4 Women's opinions on average minimum and maximum age at marriage for boys and girls by marriage cohort, 2002 IFTS

Province	Marriage Cohort	Minimum for girls	Maximum for girls	Minimum for boys	Maximum for boys
Gilan	<1980	19.5	23.3	22.8	26.8
	1980s	19.8	23.8	23.2	27.4
	1990+	20.2	24.4	24.1	28.4
West Azarbaijan	<1980	18.8	23.1	22.9	27.2
	1980s	19.1	23.5	23.0	27.7
	1990+	19.2	23.8	23.3	27.9
Sistan & Baluchistan	<1980	17.6	21.3	21.7	25.6
	1980s	17.5	20.9	21.6	25.9
	1990+	17.7	21.2	21.8	26.0
Yazd	<1980	18.5	22.4	22.6	26.9
	1980s	18.6	22.8	23.1	27.5
	1990+	19.0	23.5	23.6	28.2

that the older generation and the younger generation are presently in strong agreement about appropriate ages at marriage. The older generation does not have an expectation that their daughters should marry at very young ages. Nevertheless, the preferred marriage ages remain relatively young by international standards given the levels of education. This may partly be because work opportunities in the modern economy for young women, even young educated women, are very meagre presenting little or no alternative to relatively early marriage. Thus, unlike some countries especially in East Asia and particularly in Japan (Tsuya and Mason 1995), the fertility decline does not appear to have been related to a social change in which young women remain single longer and become involved in employment outside the household. Differences by province, on the other hand, do match the fertility differences with the exception that Yazd, again, appears to have early marriage preferences compared to the ranking of its fertility.

Relationship Between Husband and Wife[1]

Historical sources indicate that marriage between close relatives is a traditional practice in Iran (Ketabi 2000). However, studies of consanguineous marriage are limited. Using data from the 1976–1977 Iran Fertility Survey, Givens and Hirschman (1994) examined the trend and social correlates of consanguineous marriage in Iran. They found that around 40% of respondents were married to a relative, with about 24% to a near relative and 15% to a far relative. Saadat et al. (2004) conducted a national survey to investigate the prevalence and patterns of consanguinity in Iran, focusing on 12 ethnic/religious populations. The mean proportion of consanguineous marriages in the country was 38.6%, ranging from 15.9% in the northern provinces to 47% in the eastern provinces.

If the incidence of cousin marriage were to change across time, this would suggest that there were new ideas about the nature of the marriage relationship. It would suggest that family control over marriage was waning thus providing more autonomy to the younger generation. This autonomy might then transfer to changed fertility behaviour.

Tables 8.5 demonstrates the level and trend of consanguinity by province, area of residence, education, sect of religion, and ethnicity. The results in the last row of the table show that as a whole around 40% of marriages in the four provinces were consanguineous (around 21% married to first cousin and around 19% married to other relatives) and this level hardly changes across time. Around 38% of marriages for the first marriage cohort were consanguineous, the percentage increased to around 43 for the second cohort (coinciding with the Islamic revolution and the early years of the 1980s) and then declined to 39% for the third cohort. Given the changes in education level and social changes across these years, this trend suggests

[1] See Abbasi-Shavazi et al. (2008b) for a detailed analysis of consanguinity in Iran using IFTS data.

Table 8.5 Percentage of consanguinity (married to any relative) among ever-married women 15–49 by selected characteristics and marriage cohort, 2002 IFTS

Marriage cohort	<1979 (Before Islamic revolution)		1979–89 (First years of revolution and war)		1990+ (Construction and policy reforms)		Total	
Characteristics	%	*n*	%	*n*	%	*n*	%	*n*
Province								
Gilan	25.4	310	24.9	445	22.3	507	24.0	1,262
West Azarbaijan	27.3	346	38.1	473	31.1	495	32.6	1,314
Sistan and Baluchistan	78.1	220	74.8	372	79.5	427	77.4	1,019
Yazd	45.0	346	50.9	459	42.1	434	46.3	1,239
Area of residence								
Rural	42.0	597	46.8	785	47.4	986	45.8	2,368
Urban	34.2	625	39.3	964	30.7	877	35.0	2,466
Education								
Illiterate	39.5	751	48.0	623	61.0	347	46.9	1,721
Primary	37.4	349	45.4	629	40.0	619	41.5	1,597
Secondary	41.8	55	35.6	295	32.6	477	34.3	827
Diploma or higher	17.5	67	28.0	202	26.1	420	25.8	689
Sect of religion								
Sunni	53.0	297	59.6	458	59.0	549	57.8	1,304
Shiite	31.8	925	35.4	1,291	30.1	1314	32.5	3,530
Ethnicity								
Fars	49.3	431	54.0	592	43.0	584	48.7	1,607
Azari	26.2	224	37.1	339	29.7	323	31.6	886
Gilak	26.1	263	21.6	363	21.7	410	22.8	1,036
Kurd	27.6	151	39.6	190	32.9	214	33.8	555
Baluch	85.8	119	81.6	211	86.8	289	84.8	619
Total	37.9	1222	42.6	1749	39.3	1863	40.1	4,834

that cultural maintenance may have played a significant role in the persistence of traditional behaviour despite the forces of modernization.

Consanguineous marriage stands at more than 77% for all women in Sistan and Baluchistan. Despite its high level of development, marriage with a relative remains very prominent in Yazd accounting for over 46% of all marriages. On the other hand, around 33% and 24% respectively of marriages in West Azarbaijan and Gilan were consanguineous. These provinces have experienced different levels of fertility, Sistan and Baluchistan has had the highest fertility followed by West Azarbaijan and Yazd. Gilan province has one the lowest fertility in Iran (Abbasi-Shavazi et al. 2003; Abbasi-Shavazi and McDonald 2005). The trend of marriage to biological relatives in the four provinces is also mixed. Only Gilan has experienced a consistent decline in the level of consanguinity; West Azarbaijan province showed an increase during the first two periods, and then a declining trend during the last two periods while in Sistan and Baluchistan there was a slight decline (78 to 75) during the first period and then an increase to 79% during the last period. Nonetheless, the level of consanguinity has not changed in the provinces very much, and the provincial differences have been constant across cohorts.

The incidence of consanguinity is lower for women living in urban areas (around 35%) relative to those in rural areas (46%). Consanguinity has increased in rural areas across marriage cohorts but women in urban areas displayed an initial increase during the first period followed by a decline during the second period. The rise in rural areas is probably the result of selective out-migration of women more likely to have not married a relative.

There is a strong inverse relationship between women's education and consanguinity across marriage cohorts. Illiterate women were more likely than women with any other level of education to marry their relatives. As a whole, around 47% of women with no schooling had married their relatives (first or second cousins). The figures for women with primary, secondary, and diploma and higher education were around 41%, 34%, and 26%, respectively. There has been a general increase in consanguinity over time for women with no education and for those with primary education, except the last period. This is probably again the result of selection as the low education categories became much less common across time. For women with a secondary level of education, there has been a decrease in consanguinity. However, the figure for women with diploma and higher education increased from 17% to 28% and then declined to 26% by the 1990s. These results are consistent with an interpretation that, as education levels increase, each education category, particularly at the bottom and the top of the distribution, becomes increasingly more selective (compared to previous cohorts at the same education level) of women who behave in a more conservative way. For example, the very small group of highly educated women prior to 1980 (5% of all women) were likely to be less traditional in behaviour than the larger group of highly educated women after 1990 (21% of all women). If this interpretation is correct, education does not have a consistent meaning across time.

IFTS provides data on sect of religion and ethnicity. Sunni women (around 58%) were more likely to marry their relative than Shiite women (33%). There has been an increasing trend in consanguinity for Sunni women but the level of marriage to biological relatives increased for Shiite women during the first period and then declined during the last two periods. There was a variation in the level of consanguinity across cohorts among ethnic groups. Consanguinity was exceptionally high among Baluchi women, 85% of whom had married a relative. The incidence of consanguineous marriage was lower than 50% among other ethnic groups. The level of consanguinity was around 49% among Farsi speaking women followed by Kurds (34%), and Azaris (32%). Gilaki women had the lowest percentage of marriage to biological relatives (23%). These ethnic differentials in consanguinity are consistent with the findings of other studies (Saadat et al. 2004, Table 2; Abbasi-Shavazi and Sadeghi 2005:35–38; Torabi 2006).

Multivariate analysis confirmed the dominant influence of cultural variables especially ethnicity upon the incidence of consanguinity. Across time, ethnicity has remained by far the most important determinant of consanguineous marriage. In contrast, the modernization variable, education, had little significant effect upon behaviour, the effect being only for those with tertiary education (Abbasi-Shavazi et al. 2008b).

As indicated in Table 8.5, despite its very low fertility, marriage with a relative remains very prominent in Yazd accounting for over 40% of all marriages. Thus, the fertility decline has taken place while family arrangements about the nature of the marriage relationship have remained unchanged.

Attitudes About Marriage with a Relative

Table 8.6 shows percentages of ever married women 15–49 agreeing with consanguinity (marrying a relative) for both girls and boys by demographic characteristics and marriage cohort.

Table 8.6 Percentages of ever married women 15–49 agreeing with consanguineous marriage for both girls and boys by their characteristics and marriage cohort, 2002 IFTS

Marriage cohort	<1979		1979–89		1990+			
	(Before Islamic revolution)		(First years of revolution and war)		(Construction and policy reforms)		Total	
Characteristics	%	*n*	%	*n*	%	*n*	%	*n*
Province								
Gilan	10.8	310	6.6	445	8.9	507	8.5	1,262
West Azarbaijan	23.7	346	22.0	473	19.5	495	21.5	1,314
Sistan and Baluchistan	61.2	220	64.4	372	63.7	427	63.4	1,019
Yazd	27.4	346	22.0	459	16.9	434	21.7	1,239
Area of residence								
Rural	31.5	597	31.0	785	29.9	986	30.7	2,368
Urban	22.0	625	20.9	964	19.3	877	20.6	2,466
Education								
Illiterate	31.7	751	38.6	623	48.6	347	37.6	1,721
Primary	19.4	349	20.6	629	26.3	619	22.7	1,597
Secondary	10.3	55	12.5	295	15.0	477	13.8	827
Diploma or higher	7.6	67	12.5	202	11.6	420	11.5	689
Sect of religion								
Sunni	48.9	297	49.7	458	47.4	549	48.6	1,304
Shiite	17.4	925	15.0	1291	14.1	1314	15.3	3,530
Ethnicity								
Fars	30.3	431	28.0	592	20.4	584	25.8	1,607
Azari	14.4	224	16.1	339	16.9	323	15.9	886
Gilak	11.6	263	4.6	363	7.5	410	7.5	1,036
Kurd	34.7	151	29.7	190	24.6	214	29.2	555
Baluch	71.9	119	77.7	211	73.5	289	74.6	619
Current marriage								
Married a non-relative	22.3	718	20.5	941	18.3	1065	20.1	2,724
Married a relative	42.1	503	42.6	805	49.2	795	44.9	2,103
Total	26.5	1,222	25.3	1,749	24.7	1,863	25.4	4,834

Overall, around 25% of women agreed that it would be better for boys and girls to marry a relative. The differences across marriage cohorts are very small (26.5 to 24.7) indicating that women of different marriage cohorts had adopted more-or less the same attitudes to marriage to biological relatives by 2002. At the provincial level, the only major exception to this finding is for the province of Yazd where the most recent marriage cohort was much less in agreement with marriage to biological relatives than the pre-1979 marriage cohort. A strong preference for marriage to biological relatives (63%) remains prevalent only in Sistan & Baluchistan.

Women in rural areas (30%) were more in favour of marriage to biological relatives for boys and girls than those in urban areas (20%). Sunni women were more than three times more likely than Shiite women to agree with marriage to biological relatives and the ethnic variation in attitudes toward marriage to biological relatives was relatively similar to behaviour. Around 75% of Baluchi speaking women were in favour of consanguinity while only 7.5% of Gilaki women reported that it would be better if girls/boys marry a relative. Not unexpectedly, those who had themselves married a relative were much more likely to agree with marriage to biological relatives for boys and girls (45%) than those who had not married a relative (20%).

The pattern of attitudes by education across marriage cohorts is very interesting. It shows that the percentage that favoured marriage with a relative increased for all education categories from the first cohort to the third cohort. This means, effectively, that within each education level, younger women were more likely than older women to favour marriage with a relative. As argued above, this may mean that education does not have a consistent association with modern thought across time. As more women become educated, each education category becomes relatively less modern in its thought compared to the same education category in earlier periods. The increase in agreement with consanguinity across time within each education category is reconciled with the absence of an increase for all women by recognising the impact of the compositional shift of the population by education. If the pre-1979 cohort had had the same educational composition as the 1990+ cohort, agreement with consanguinity for the pre-1979 group would have been 39.5% rather than 26.5% actually observed. For the 1979–1989 cohort, agreement would have been 31.6% if their educational composition had been the same as the 1990+ cohort compared with the actual level of 25.3%. This is all suggestive that, as women in a cohort shift upwards in education, some may retain aspects of their cultural beliefs rather than adopting the views of their new educational category as held by the previous cohort.

While the ‘no difference’ category makes explanation tentative, it is interesting that attitudes to marriage with a relative seem to be running ahead of behaviour. Thus, there is some evidence that behaviour may be modified somewhat in this regard in the future reflecting some shift away from traditional approaches to marriage.

Our analysis of attitudes (Abbasi-Shavazi et al. 2008b), an indicator of future change, again confirmed the dominance of cultural factors. Being of the Shiite sect was a strong predictor of opposition to consanguineous marriage among women who themselves had married a relative. Furthermore, there was evidence that growing opposition to consanguineous marriage was associated with ethnicity with opposition being higher among women who themselves had married a relative in ethnic groups where consanguineous marriage was less common. Consistent with the theory of idealized morality (McDonald 1994), the effects of education (modernization) were filtered through the cultural variables, sect of Islam and ethnicity.

Co-Residence After Marriage

With the notable exception of Yazd, a similar conclusion can be drawn in relation to place of residence following the marriage. The proportions of couples that lived with the extended family have not changed across time in three of the four provinces (Table 8.7).

In Yazd, there was a fairly substantial movement away from living with the extended family after marriage but this may well be related to the prevalence of long distance migration in Yazd Province, especially to the city of Yazd. To explain fertility decline, we are looking for features that are replicated across all four provinces. Thus, again, changes in family organization do not seem to have been important.[2] Abbasi-Shavazi and Askari-Nodoushan (2005) examined the impact of co-residence after marriage on fertility in Yazd province. Contrary to expectations,

Table 8.7 Percentages distribution of women by co-residence over 2 years after marriage, province and marriage cohorts, 2002 IFTS

		Co-residence				
Province	Marriage cohort	Woman's relative	Woman and husband's relative	Husband's relative	None	Number of women
Gilan	<1980	5.8	4.2	59.4	30.7	363
	1980s	8.4	3.1	61.0	27.5	392
	1990+	9.4	4.7	57.6	28.3	507
West Azarbaijan	<1980	2.5	7.1	71.3	19.1	389
	1980s	3.6	6.2	79.1	11.2	429
	1990+	3.2	5.7	76.9	14.2	496
Sistan & Baluchistan	<1980	20.2	6.0	45.1	28.7	255
	1980s	21.7	5.4	39.3	33.6	336
	1990+	24.9	7.9	42.1	25.1	428
Yazd	<1980	12.8	4.4	55.3	27.6	428
	1980s	8.0	1.7	48.5	41.7	376
	1990+	19.2	1.8	26.2	52.8	435

[2] The question asked if the couple lived for at least one month with one of their husband's or their own relatives after marriage. If so, then they should choose options one to three accordingly, otherwise they should choose the 'none' category. Thus, the high prevalence of living with relatives shown in the table does not necessarily imply a long period of co-residence with relatives after marriage.

they concluded that women who were co-residing with their relative after marriage were likely to have lower fertility than those who were not living with their relatives after marriage. They concluded that co-residence was not related to the rapid changes that have taken place in fertility attitudes and behaviours while traditional elements of family have experienced continuity and change in recent years. Thus, the sharp fertility decline in Iran cannot be explained by changes in family as the rapid fall has not been accompanied by rapid transformations of traditional elements of family life, and contrary to the prediction of some scholars, no linear convergence has been observed towards the Western nuclear family in Iran (see also: Abbasi-Shavazi and McDonald 2007; Abbasi-Shavazi et al. 2008a).

Preference for Early Marriage or Continued Education for Girls

Table 8.8 shows that, across all provinces and across all marriage cohorts, there is a strong preference that girls continue their education in preference to marrying early. The majority (more than 70%) of women of the three marriage cohorts preferred education over marriage for girls, the exception being Yazd where women expressed more conservative views toward marriage. This indicates a valuing of education for girls despite the fact that this does not flow through to high rates of employment prior to marriage.

The pattern seems to be that it is good for girls to be educated and this has flowed through to substantial increases in levels of education for girls, but, to this point in time, it has been mainly education for marriage and family rather than education for employment. Nevertheless, the strong preference for education for girls has had its outcome and may have had an impact on the status of women

Table 8.8 Percentage of women preferring continuation of education rather than early marriage for a girl and their reasons by province and marriage cohorts, 2002 IFTS

Province	Marriage cohort	Prefer continuing education for girls	Distribution of women by reason: Better opportunity for marriage	For child rearing in future	Finding an appropriate job	Other	Number of women
Gilan	<1980	69.6	12.2	7.1	68.1	12.6	363
	1980s	73.5	13.9	8.6	69.7	7.7	392
	1990+	71.8	16	12.1	62.5	9.4	507
West Azarbaijan	<1980	76.9	15.8	8.2	70.6	5.3	429
	1980s	79.4	12.5	9.1	69.1	9.2	496
	1990+	81	18.5	11.2	62.3	8	255
Sistan & Baluchistan	<1980	71.2	12.3	18.8	61.7	7.2	428
	1980s	75.4	10.8	19.9	64.1	5.2	428
	1990+	73.1	11.3	24.1	60.4	4.2	376
Yazd	<1980	54.5	21.3	33.1	42	3.5	363
	1980s	53.2	38	31.7	26.9	3.5	392
	1990+	65.2	41	27.5	28.4	3.1	507

within the marriage. This in turn, as argued above, may lead to lower fertility. Interestingly, Yazd, a conservative province, maintains relatively conservative attitudes in this regard despite the fact that its education levels are actually higher than in any of the other four provinces.

Overall, as indicated, education is valued in the society even among older cohorts who were either illiterate or less educated. This may be considered as a measure of ideational change in the society as there are few generational differences in the provinces under scrutiny, particularly in West Azarbaijan and Sistan & Baluchistan.

Women who believed that girls should marry early rather than continue their education, had more-or-less traditional gender values. Most of them indicated that girls should marry early either because they may not have the opportunity to marry later, or they considered that the main task of women is housekeeping. However, one third of these women, again, thought that girls could continue their education after marriage.

The majority (around 70%) of women who preferred education over early marriage for girls believed that girls should continue their education to find an appropriate job in the future (Table 8.8). As indicated earlier, female employment is very low in Iran (around 12%). However, with the rising of education levels, occupational aspirations of girls have risen and it is possible that Iranian society will experience major changes with regard to women's employment in the future. The percentages of women who considered girls should be educated in order to find a job in the future in the three provinces of Gilan, West Azarbaijan, and Sistan & Baluchistan were high and at a similar level. On the other hand, compared to work, women in Yazd placed more emphasis on enhancement of marriage and family outcomes as reasons for girl's to pursue education, and this pattern was more evident for the more recent cohorts compared to the oldest cohort. In Yazd, there may have been an expectation of the 'proper' answer to this question but this in itself has meaning. The expression of more conservative attitudes by women in Yazd is consistent across all indicators.

Family Planning and Fertility Behaviour

Turning now to more direct measures of fertility behaviour, women were asked how long after marriage conceived their first pregnancy. The results show little evidence of an impact on fertility of a change in the interval between marriage and first birth. The interval is short in general and highest in Sistan & Baluchistan which has the highest level of fertility. The longest first birth interval relates to the cohort that had the highest fertility – the oldest cohort in Sistan & Baluchistan.

The interval between marriage and first birth decreased for all marriage cohorts in all provinces except in Yazd where the interval increased for the recent cohort. This is consistent with the findings of Rindfuss and Morgan (1983) who found shortening of birth interval in other Asian countries. The decline of birth intervals from the marriage cohorts of 1976–1980 to 1981–1985 was noticeable. For example, in Gilan, women who married before the 1980s, on average had their birth within the first 10 months after marriage but it decreased to 8.4 months for those who married during the 1980s. The decline was sharper for women in West Azarbaijan where the figure decreased from 13 months to around 10 months, and for women in Sistan and Baluchistan where the fall was from around 18 months to 14 months. This is consistent with the rise of fertility immediately before and after the revolution in these provinces (Abbasi-Shavazi 2000). Marriage and childbearing were encouraged during the first decade after the revolution, legal mean age at marriage for both girls and boys decreased, and marriage was considered as a way of keeping young boys and girls faithful to traditional family values rather than being corrupted by 'Western values'. The other point to be noted here is that having the first birth is very important for families in Iran and couples are expected to have their first child early in their life to fulfil societal and familial expectations.

Women were asked whether they were using contraceptives before their first pregnancy. The results (Fig. 8.1) show that practice of birth control before pregnancy has changed across cohorts with younger cohorts in Gilan and Yazd being more likely to use contraceptives before their first birth than older cohorts. As shown, in Gilan, the percentage of women who used contraception before their first pregnancy increased from 3.6% for marriage cohort 1976–1980 to 7.4% for those married during the late 1980s. This figures increased significantly to around 17% and 24% respectively for the two marriage cohorts 1991–1995 and 1996+. Similar trend is found for Yazd but the figure for the latest cohort increased to around 35%.

While this change does not seem to have had much impact on the interval from marriage to the first birth (except in Yazd where first birth interval has increased slightly), it may be a precursor to future changes. Another analysis in this book shows an emerging strong use of contraception before the first birth in Tehran City (not included in the 2002 IFTS survey). We have analysed the use of birth control prior to

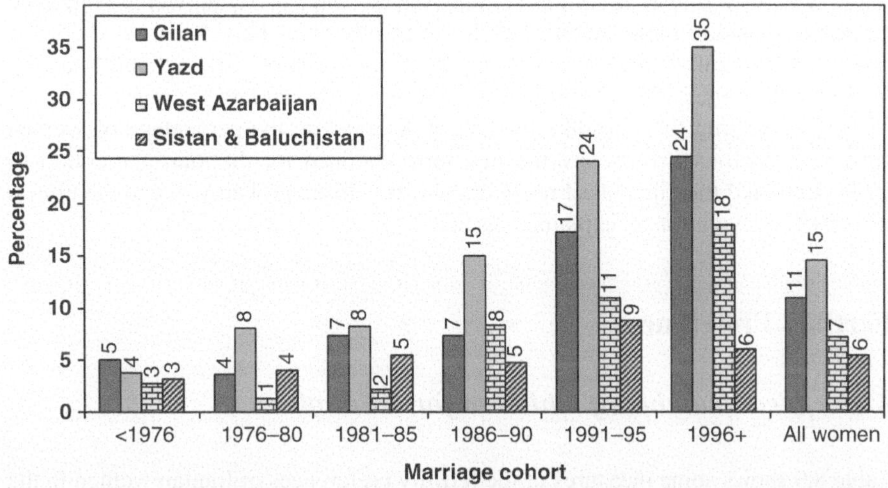

Fig. 8.1 Percentage of women by use of contraceptives before the first pregnancy by marriage cohort and province, 2002 IFTS

first pregnancy in more detail (Abbasi-Shavazi et al. 2009). We conceptualised family change as structural change and, in turn, structure as produced from the interplay of available schema and resources (Sewell 1992, 2005). Compatible with this framework are two contrasting explanations for the increase in birth control use immediately following marriage. The first, the conjugal marriage explanation, posits that this innovative behaviour signals the emergence of a new marriage form, the conjugal marriage. This new marriage form is characterized by a focus on strong emotional bonds between husband and wife, egalitarian values and a weakened gender division of labour. The force driving marriage change in this direction is globalisation and westernisation, and available Western schema supportive of individualism and self-actualisation (Goode 1963; also see Thornton 2001, 2005). The alternative explanation, one more consistent with evidence examined here, stressed that an idealized family morality (McDonald 1994) supported by powerful institutions, and personified in Iran by the state/religion nexus, provide powerful resources supporting an Iranian–Islamic family schema. The state is focused on encouraging early marriage and provides resources for doing so. As a result individuals turn to birth control early in marriage to conform to early marriage expectations while postponing parenthood. This explanation sees the new behaviour as conservative, maintaining relatively early marriage. A new behaviour, birth control use, can be seen as strengthening and cementing the traditional schema because contraceptive use is interpreted and motivated by the traditional schema. This schema was legitimated by religious leaders' reinterpretations of family planning as fundamentally Islamic (and not as "originating in modern Western society") (Hoodfar and Assadpour 2000:28).

Delay of the first birth with marriage in combination with high education levels of women could promote the employment of married women. On the other hand, job opportunities for young married women may be restricted because of within-cohort competition for the very large cohorts born in the early 1980s. Competition with young men in the labour market may see the entry of young women into paid employment being more muted than it might otherwise have been. At the same time, employment difficulties for young men may promote delayed child-bearing leading to an expectation of further falls in cross-sectional fertility rates.

It is interesting that, in Gilan and West Azarbaijan, the percentage of women who used contraceptive before the first birth declined for the marriage cohort of 1976–1980 and then increased for later cohorts. This is probably due to the effects of the 1979 revolution as explained earlier.

Fertility Preferences

Mean Ideal Number of Children for a Couple

Table 8.9 shows some measures of the fertility preferences of Iranian women in the four provinces. The numbers desired at the time of marriage show an expected fall across time. However, the fall is much more muted than the actual fertility decline

Table 8.9 Mean number of desired children at the time of marriage and survey, and mean number of children considered as too high and too low, by province and marriage cohort, 2002 IFTS

Province	Marriage cohort	Number of children wanted at time of marriage	Currently appropriate number of children for a couple	How many children are too many?	How many children are too few?
Gilan	<1980	2.9	2.0	4.5	1.4
	1980s	2.4	1.9	4.5	1.6
	1990+	1.9	2.0	4.1	1.4
West Azarbaijan	<1980	3.4	2.5	4.9	1.8
	1980s	2.6	2.2	4.3	1.3
	1990+	2.0	2.1	4.2	1.5
Sistan & Baluchistan	<1980	5.4	4.1	6.8	2.0
	1980s	4.4	3.2	7.0	2.7
	1990+	3.8	3.7	6.5	2.7
Yazd	<1980	3.9	2.5	5.3	1.4
	1980s	3.2	2.3	5.0	1.3
	1990+	2.4	2.2	4.7	1.2

because the earlier marriage cohorts state numbers much lower than the numbers that they actually had. This can be interpreted to mean that:

1. The older cohorts had many children that they did not want suggesting an unmet need for family planning. or
2. The older cohorts have rationalized their response to this question in the light of the subsequent fall in fertility.

Whichever meaning is taken, the older generation is expressing that the number of children that they had was too high, and this is confirmed by the fact that the numbers they give as 'too many' tend to be below the number they actually had themselves. This means that the older generation today would be supportive of the smaller family ideals of the younger generation. This is confirmed by their statement of the number of children that is most appropriate for couples today which is generally similar to that of younger cohorts. For younger cohorts (married since 1980), the average number wanted at marriage is similar to the number considered to be appropriate for couples today suggesting that, on average, couples are having the number they would like to have.

Even for the most recent marriage cohort, fertility preferences in Sistan & Baluchistan remain considerably higher than in the other three provinces suggesting that the higher fertility in that province is likely to remain evident for some time. Higher fertility in Sistan & Baluchistan should be interpreted according to the cultural and social-economic context of the province. Sistan & Baluchistan is the least developed province in the country. The majority of the people are Sunni sects of Islam who mainly speak Baluchi. Although both ethnicity and religion may have some influence on fertility, it is hard to control and separate the impact of ethnicity/religion on fertility, even using multivariate analysis. The Baluchi in Sistan &

Baluchistan have a considerable degree of contact with the Baluchi in Pakistan's province of Baluchistan with cross-border marriages being common (see Chapter 3). Among Pakistan's Baluchi, however, the education level of young women remains low and family planning knowledge is not as advanced as it is across the border in Iran. Hence, the cross-border influence may keep the fertility level of Iran's Baluchi higher than it would otherwise have been as wives tend to move to the husband's household.

Distribution of the Ideal Number of Children for a Couple

Table 8.10 shows the distribution of women by their preferred ideal number of children for a couple at the time of the survey. Three main findings emerge. First, in all provinces, except in Sistan & Baluchistan, the majority of women indicated that two children is the ideal number for a couple today. In Sistan & Baluchistan only 40% to 45% of each marriage cohort considered two children as ideal while 40% believed that four children or more would be ideal for a couple. Second, there are no considerable variations in ideal family sizes across marriage cohorts, particularly in Gilan and West Azarbaijan provinces. Third, relatively high percentages of all marriage cohorts in Gilan preferred one child as the ideal number of children for a couple. This is very high for the Iranian context and, indeed, for any context, and may have implications for the future of fertility in Iran.

If women indicated one child, or two-or-more children as an ideal number of children for a couple, they were then asked the reason why they prefer *"N"* number of children as an ideal number for a couple. Respondents were given 13 options, and were asked to identify these options according to three priorities. Women who preferred one child overwhelmingly referred to rising family costs as the main

Table 8.10 Percentage distribution of women by currently ideal number of children, province and marriage cohorts, 2002 IFTS

Provinces	Marriage cohorts	Ideal number of children for a couple				Number of women
		1	2	3	4+	
Gilan	<1980	17.9	70.5	9.4	2.2	363
	1980s	18.5	74.3	5.2	2.0	392
	1990+	22.4	71.5	5.0	1.2	507
West Azarbaijan	<1980	4.0	70.4	17.1	8.5	389
	1980s	5.7	73.0	14.9	6.4	429
	1990+	10.3	73.2	14.5	2.0	496
Sistan & Baluchistan	<1980	2.5	39.9	14.5	43.0	255
	1980s	2.0	43.0	15.3	39.8	336
	1990+	3.6	46.9	11.8	37.6	428
Yazd	<1980	2.7	60.8	23.3	13.1	428
	1980s	3.0	68.9	21.2	6.9	376
	1990+	7.2	73.8	14.3	4.6	435

reason for preferring such a low ideal family size with quality of children as a secondary reason (results not shown here). The pattern of responses was similar for those women who thought two children was the ideal number of children for a couple with rising family costs being by far the most prominent reason for the choice of this ideal (around 60%). Quality of children (measured by '*to rear children better*' and '*to provide better facilities for children*') was the other important reason expressed for indicating two children as ideal. Reasons such as child survival, parent's welfare and progress and provision of a sibling were also expressed, but by relatively small numbers of women. For the relatively small proportions who stated four or more children as ideal, the reason that children would look after their parents in old age also emerged.

In summary, the interesting finding from this section is the ideational change in Iranian society evident by the fact that ideal family size/fertility is similar among young and older cohorts. It is also notable that even those who had higher fertility considered two children as the ideal number of children for a couple, but that in Gilan, there has been a relatively high preference for one child even among the previous cohorts. The percentage of those who preferred one child in Gilan has increased from 18% to 22.5% for the recent cohort. The figures for other provinces are considerably lower than Gilan but there has been an increasing trend across cohorts. Overwhelmingly, low expressed ideals were associated with economic motivations related to the perceived costs of children.

Attitudes Toward Childbearing/Value of Children

Table 8.11 shows the distribution of women agreeing with different statements representing various (traditional versus liberal) views regarding children. The results are shown for different cohorts of women in each province. For example, the first column describes attitudes of women towards the statement 'Parents should have many children for their aging time'. Around 27% of women in Gilan who married before 1980s agreed with this statement. The figure declined to 16% and 14% for the next two cohorts indicating that this attitude has shifted downwards across cohorts. Similar results are shown for women in West Azarbaijan and Yazd with downward trend. However, as expected, women in Sistan and Baluchistan have more conservative attitudes towards childbearing, as 56% of older cohorts agreed with the statement, and the figure declined to 48% for the next two cohorts. The next item reveals women's attitudes towards the statement 'Having many children is an obstacle to the parents' interests'. This is considered as a liberal view which is an indication of the costs of childbearing for parents. As indicated, the vast majority of women in all provinces agreed with this statement. In Gilan around 89% of the older cohort and 90% of the two recent cohorts agreed with the statement. In West Azarbaijan and Yazd also between 83% and 86% of women of different cohorts agreed with this statement. Similarly, the vast majority of women agreed with the following two statements 'Having many children creates psychological stress for parents' and

Table 8.11 Percentage of women agreeing with various statements on childbearing and value of children by marriage cohorts and province, 2002 IFTS

Province	Marriage Cohort	Parents should have many children for their aging time	Having many children is an obstacle to the parents' interests	Having many children will increase the family's income	Having many children is a good help in house keeping	Having many children creates psychological stress for parents	Parents cannot properly raise many children	Having many children does not affect their education level	Having many children creates financial pressure on the family	If people had more income, they would have more children	A couple's independence increases as the number of their children increases	Birth control is an interference in God's affairs	Parents feel alive after death when they have many children	Having many children increases family and ethnic power	Having many children increases family and ethnic power
Gilan	<1980	22.7	88.9	15	26.7	96.1	89.7	13.6	97.5	20.2	16	28.6	23.9	15.9	363
	1980s	16.6	90.2	11.7	17.6	97.9	93	11.2	97.4	15.7	11.2	21.5	15	10.1	392
	1990+	14.3	91.3	11.7	22.8	97.4	94	13.1	96.4	17.3	10.2	15.6	15.7	8.6	507
	Total	17.4	90.3	12.6	22.3	97.2	92.5	12.7	97	17.6	12.1	21.2	17.8	11.2	1,262
West Azarbaijan	<1980	25.1	85.7	18.6	31.2	94.7	88.5	17.7	97.6	16.4	17.2	27.4	27.3	29.1	389
	1980s	24.2	86.5	19.3	28.3	96.2	91.9	14.1	96.9	16.3	10.6	24.1	22.6	25.2	429
	1990+	19.7	86.5	18.5	26.9	96.6	93.4	15.9	97.3	14	12.2	18.6	20.4	20.9	496
	Total	22.8	86.3	18.8	28.6	95.9	91.4	15.8	97.2	15.4	13.2	23	23.2	24.8	1,314
Sistan & Baluchistan	<1980	55.9	71.8	47.3	59.3	87.9	85.3	34.4	88.7	43	42.5	47.7	46.4	46.9	255
	1980s	48.3	70.2	41.9	56.3	88	85.3	33.8	90.6	39.1	31.3	36.4	39.3	41.7	336
	1990+	47.8	70.5	38.9	49	86.7	83.9	31.8	90.1	39.2	30.5	40.2	38	41.7	428
	Total	50	70.7	41.9	53.9	87.4	84.7	33.1	89.9	40.1	33.7	40.8	40.5	43	1,019
Yazd	<1980	29.8	87.7	14.7	29.3	96.4	93.3	9.6	97.3	18.9	18.7	36.5	22.6	15	428
	1980s	25.6	82.3	14.5	21.4	93.6	93	12.1	97.5	18.2	15	31.6	19.6	13.1	376
	1990+	19.5	83	9.9	21.6	97	96.4	7.2	97.8	14.1	10	23.2	15.6	10	435
	Total	25	84.4	13	24.2	95.7	94.3	9.5	97.5	17	14.6	30.4	19.3	12.7	1,239

'Having many children creates financial pressure on the family', as more than 95% of women of all marriage cohorts in Gilan, Yazd and West Azarbaijan, and around 88% of women in Sistan and Baluchistan agreed with these statements.

In general, women in all provinces, except Sistan & Baluchistan, expressed liberal views about childbearing. For example, the majority of women disagreed with the following statements regarded as traditional values:

- Parents should have many children for their old age.
- Having many children will increase family income.
- Having many children is a good help in housekeeping.
- Having many children does not affect their education level.
- If people had more income they would have more children.
- The couple's independence increases as the number of their children increases.
- Birth control is an interference in God's affairs.
- Parents feel alive after death when they have many children.
- Having many children increases family and ethnic power.

On the other hand, the vast majority of women agreed with the following "liberal" statements:

- Having many children is an obstacle for the parents' interests
- Having many children creates psychological stress for parents.
- Parents cannot properly raise many children.
- Having many children creates financial pressure for the family.

The other interesting finding is that there were not many differences between the marriage cohorts but, where there were differences, the direction was towards more liberal values among the more recent marriage cohorts. Only in Sistan & Baluchistan were conservative views expressed by relatively large numbers but, even in this province, the emphasis on liberal views was higher than on the conservative. For example, most women in Sistan & Baluchistan disagreed that 'having many children would increase the family's income'.

Consistent with the stated reasons for low fertility ideals, there was strong agreement with all statements that expressed the view that children were an economic disadvantage and strong disagreement with statements that they were an economic advantage. However, non-economic values related to small family size also received substantial agreement including those related to the level of stress upon parents, the obstacle that children present to parents pursuing their own interests and the raising of 'quality' children. The traditional views that birth control is an interference in God's affairs, that many children represent greater power for the family or the ethnic group, or that more children means 'life after death' were supported by only about one fifth of respondents in Gilan, Yazd and West Azarbaijan. Support was stronger for these statements in Sistan & Baluchistan but was still lower than 50%.

The overall impression from these results is that a norm of low fertility has spread across Iran and it has been adopted by both older and younger generations. The older generation who themselves had very high fertility are now almost equal in their strong support of a low fertility norm with the younger generation. The significance of this norm is evidenced by the fact that it is justified by Iranians using economic, soical and psychological reasons and beacuse Iranians provide strongly negative evaluation of the impacts of high fertility on both the children and the parents. Furthermore, the expression of the norm in terms of attitudes and values is consistently interpreted across the provinces included in the survey.

It is also interesting that women do not think that increased governmental financial support would encourage couples to have more children. More than 70% of women in Gilan, more than 80% in West Azarbaijan and Yazd, and more than 60% of women in Sistan & Baluchistan disagreed with the statement that higher government financial support would encourage families to have more children. On the other hand, they believed that government regulations and punishments for having more than two children would encourage families to control their fertility (Abbasi-Shavazi et al. 2003).

Gender Roles

Table 8.12 shows the percentages of women who agreed with a range of statements about employment of women outside the home. In general, the expressed attitudes indicate much more support for the employment of women outside of the home than is actually the case at present. Again, it seems that attitudes are running ahead of behaviour suggesting considerable potential for future change. Women in all four provinces were especially likely to agree that women should work for financial autonomy or to support their family financially. The economic motivation for social change is again prominent. However, except in Yazd, a majority also considered that women should work outside the home for the social participation that this would entail. Conversely, only 30–40% of women agreed that 'a woman should not work outside the home, her duty is housekeeping' and 'employed women cannot rear their children well'. In general, these attitudes did not vary much across provinces or across generations.

Other data from IFTS (results not shown here) show that decisions within marriage about purchase of food, household equipment or gold/jewels tend to be cooperative decisions of the husband and the wife and that the cooperative model is more prominent among the more recent marriage cohorts than among earlier cohorts. Respondents were also asked if they had ever been beaten by their husbands.[3] Again, across marriage cohorts from older to younger, there was a considerable

[3]The question by asking 'ever' would be answered in the affirmative by women who had only one experience during their marriage. The impression gained from the responses may tend therefore to exaggerate the incidence of violence within marriage. Nevertheless, there were substantial falls in the reported incidence from older to younger cohorts as would be expected if levels of gender equity were improving in association with increased levels of education.

Table 8.12 Percentage of women agreeing with various statements about employment of women outside the home by marriage cohorts and province, 2002 IFTS

Province	Marriage cohort	A woman should not work outside home, her duty is housekeeping	Employed women cannot rear their children very well	Employed women have fewer children	Women must be employed for financial autonomy	Women should not work outside home like men	Women should work outside home to support family financially	Women should work outside home for social participation	Number of women
Gilan	<1980	41.1	38	83.8	79	41.3	85.1	59.1	363
	1980s	31.4	28.9	73.7	73.9	39.5	84.5	53.7	392
	1990+	31.7	31.7	73	70.3	37.1	80.6	54.9	507
	Total	34.3	32.6	76.3	73.9	39.1	83.1	55.7	1,262
West Azarbaijan	<1980	44.9	41.6	69.3	75.2	43.9	71.3	64.9	389
	1980s	40.4	36.9	60.1	74.1	41.5	75.1	64.7	429
	1990+	40.1	34.5	59	68.3	41.7	66.8	60	496
	Total	41.6	37.4	62.4	72.3	42.3	70.9	63	1,314
Sistan & Baluchistan	<1980	42.1	45.4	78.6	76.7	39.9	73.8	63.6	255
	1980s	36	35.7	73.5	74.6	34.3	69.2	62.8	336
	1990+	37.8	35.8	70.1	67	39.2	68.3	60.6	428
	Total	38.3	38.1	73.3	71.9	37.8	70	62.1	1,019
Yazd	<1980	40.8	44.3	80.2	75.8	48.4	66.3	48.4	428
	1980s	33	38.3	69.1	70.4	42.1	59.1	45.1	376
	1990+	22.8	30.8	61.8	66.2	31	68.2	45.1	435
	Total	32.2	37.8	70.4	70.8	40.4	64.7	46.2	1,239

shift away from women reporting that they had been beaten. There was also a shift away from women reporting that they had a 'general fear' of their husband. All of these changes can be interpreted as indicating an increase in the level of gender equity in couple relationships within the family. Other questions that were more related to the external role of women, especially questions related to the woman's freedom of movement outside the household, showed less change across the generations. Nevertheless, among the most recent marriage cohort, only 35–40% of married women in Gilan and Yazd say that they must ask their husband's permission before going to a health centre or doctor, and only 14% (Gilan) and 33% (Yazd) are actually accompanied when they go to the health centre or to the doctor. The results for these measures of freedom of movement were much more conservative for West Azerbaijan and Sistan & Baluchistan. The relationship between women's autonomy and reproductive behavior will be analysed in detail in the next chapter.

Conclusion and Discussion

This chapter set out to provide a cohort perspective on the changes in fertility, family behaviours and attitudes in the four selected provinces of Iran. As discussed in Chapter 5, the task of explanation of the substantial decline in fertility in Iran and in each of the four provinces becomes largely a question of why fertility within marriage has fallen. Clearly, a very substantial increase in the use of fertility control methods has been the immediate cause of the decline of fertility in marriage especially in the 1990s. However, the commencement of the fertility decline preceded the re-establishment of the nation's family planning program in 1989. This gives rise to the hypothesis that social and economic change and associated changes in attitudes and values may have precipitated the fall in fertility and increased the demand for family planning services. This chapter provides an assessment of the association between the fertility trend and the transformation of attitudes and values toward family and fertility.

Different periods of social change represented by the three time periods of marriage were used to study these changes in Iran: prior to the 1980s, during the 1980s, and during the 1990s. The result has been a complex mosaic of individual and family change and persistence in the various provinces. The most important individual change in recent decades is the increased level of education across cohorts stimulated by the egalitarian nature of the revolution. There was a significant shift from illiteracy and low levels of education among older cohorts towards much higher levels of education for younger cohorts in all of the provinces under scrutiny. Education brings with it the confidence to hold and express one's own views and increased ability to engage with the modern world and its ideas. There would seem to be little argument that the more liberal attitudes and values expressed by women in the IFTS study were related to this trend in education levels. Nevertheless, in most cases, women from the older generations also expressed relatively liberal values and attitudes to questions about numbers of children. Thus, it has to be argued that a pervasive low fertility norm has swept Iran taking with it all generations and all provinces. There remain differences between provinces but the strong expectation is that provincial differences will diminish and this is already evident in recent fertility trends. Economic motivations for changed values in relation to numbers of children or to work of women outside the home were very strongly expressed everywhere. Thus, there is strong support for the hypothesis that fertility decline has been driven by a desire for economic improvement at the household level perhaps with a reduced capacity to achieve this end. What is all the more interesting is the notion that this economic motivation arose at the heart of the early years of the Islamic revolution. The egalitarian nature of the revolution and its concern with the improvement of health services, education and living standards for all appears to have engendered economic aspirations and value changes that extended beyond the immediate aims of the revolution.

At the level of the family, several dimensions of family life have remained fairly constant, while others have changed dramatically. Fertility behaviour and attitudes of women have changed across birth and marriage cohorts over the last two decades. The ideal number of children has declined considerably across cohorts and in all provinces, even among those older cohorts who have had higher fertility. A preference for two children is common in all provinces. The relatively high prevalence of 'one child' as an ideal number of children for couples in Gilan is very interesting and has many policy implications for the future of fertility in Iran. The timing of marriage has also shifted towards higher ages, particularly for girls. There is considerable shift in women's attitudes towards girl's marriage, as women of all cohorts prefer their daughters (or girls in general) to continue their education rather than marrying earlier.

Change within the family has tended to be stronger at the level of the individual couple. This includes decisions about the numbers of children that they have and attitudes about gender roles within the couple relationship. As attention shifts from the internal or intimate to the external or public aspects of family, change becomes more muted. Marriage with relatives remains common and there has been little change across time. Married women still lead relatively restricted lives and are still largely 'subject' to their husbands in their public lives, and actual participation in work outside of the home remains low. However, in all of these public dimensions of family, attitudes have shifted and are running ahead of behaviour. Change in the external dimensions of the institution of the family remains relatively constrained because of its public nature; at the private or intimate level, change has been more possible.

In summary, fertility decline in Iran appears to have been driven by rising economic aspirations leading to the inculcation across Iran of a small family size norm. The rapid fall of fertility was then facilitated by increased levels of education, greater gender equity within the husband–wife relationship and by the provision by the Iranian Government of affordable and reliable access to family planning through the country's extensive public health system.

References

Abbasi-Shavazi MJ (2000) Effects of marital fertility and nuptiality on fertility transition in the Islamic Republic of Iran. Working Papers in Demography, No. 84, The Australian National University, Canberra

Abbasi-Shavazi MJ, Askari-Nodoushan A (2005) Family changes and fertility decline in Iran: case study in Yazd province, [Persian]. J Soc Sci 25:45–75

Abbasi-Shavazi MJ, McDonald P (2005) National and Provincial-Level Fertility Trends in Iran, 1972–2000. Working Paper in Demography No. 94. Australian National University, Canberra

Abbasi-Shavazi MJ, McDonald P (2007) Family change in Iran: religion, revolution, and the state. In: Jayakody R, Thornton A, Axinn W (eds) International family change: ideational perspectives. Taylor and Francis Group, LLC, Boca Raton, FL, pp 177–198

Abbasi-Shavazi MJ, Sadeghi R (2005) Ethnicity and family patterns in Iran [Persian]. Women Stud [Pazhuhis-i zanan] 3(1):25–47

Abbasi-Shavazi MJ, McDonald P, Hosseini-Chavoshi M (2008a) Social change and the family in post-revolutionary Iran. In: Kathryn M Yount, Hoda Rashad (eds) Family ties and ideals: portraits of continuity and change in Egypt, Iran, and Tunisia. Taylor & Francis Group, LLC, Routledge, pp 217–235

Abbasi-Shavazi MJ, McDonald P, Hosseini-Chavoshi M (2008b) Modernization and the cultural practice of consanguineous marriage in Iran. J Biosoc Sci 40(4):911–933

Abbasi-Shavazi MJ, Morgan P, McDonald P, Hosseini-Chavoshi M (2009) Family change and continuity in Iran: contraceptive use before first pregnancy. J Marriage Fam [forthcoming]

Abbasi-Shavazi MJ, McDonald P, Hosseini-Chavoshi M (2003) Changes in family, fertility behavior and attitudes in Iran. Working Paper in Demography No. 88, Australian National University, Canberra

Abbasi-Shavazi MJ, Mehryar A, Jones G, McDonald P (2002) Revolution, war and modernization: population policy and fertility change in Iran. J Popul Res 19(1):25–46

Axinn WG, Thornton A (1993) Mothers, children, and cohabitation: the intergenerational effects of attitudes and behavior. Am Sociol Rev 58:233–246

Givens PB, Hirschman C (1994) Modernization and consanguineous marriage in Iran. J Marriage Fam 56 (November), 820–834

Goode WJ (1963) World revolution and family patterns. Free Press, New York

Hoodfar H, Assadpour S (2000) The politics of population policy in the Islamic Republic of Iran. Stud Fam Plann 31(1):19–34

Ketabi A (2000) Marriage with close relatives in ancient Iran [Perisan]. J Soc Sci 16:167–192

McDonald P (1994) Families in developing countries: Idealised morality and theories of family change. In Cho, L. & Yada, M. (eds) Tradition and Change in the Asian Family. East-West Center, Honolulu, pp. 19–28

Morgan SP, Waite LJ (1987) Parenthood and the attitudes of young adults. Am Sociol Rev 52:541–547

Rindfuss RR, Morgan SP (1983) Marriage, sex, and the first birth interval: The quiet revolution in Asia. Population and Development Review, 9:259–278

Saadat M, Ansari-Lari M, Farhud DD (2004) Consanguineous marriage in Iran. Annals of Human Biology 31(2):263–269

Sewell WH (1992) A theory of structure: Duality, agency, and transformation. Am J Sociology 98:1–29

Sewell WH (2005) Logics of history. Chicago: University of Chicago Press

Thornton A (2001) The developmental paradigm, reading history sideways, and family change. Demography 38(4):449–467

Thornton A (2005) Reading history sideways. Chicago: University of Chicago Press

Thornton A, Chang JS, Lin HS (1994) From arranged marriage to love match. In: Thornton A, Lin H (eds) Social change and the family in Taiwan. University of Chicago Press, Chicago, IL, pp 148–177

Thornton A (1994) Truncation bias. In: Thornton A, Lin H (eds) Social change and the family in Taiwan. University of Chicago Press, Chicago, IL, pp 148–177

Thornton A, Lin H (1994) Social change and the family in Taiwan. University of Chicago Press, Chicago, IL

Thornton A (1989) Changing attitudes toward family issues in the United States. J Marriage Fam 51:873–893

Thornton A, Young-Demarco L (2001) Four decades of trends in attitudes toward family issues in the United States: the 1960s through 1990s. J Marriage Fam 63:1009–1037

Thornton A, Freedman D (1982) Changing attitudes toward marriage and single life. Fam Plann Perspect 14(6):297–303

Torabi F (2006) Social, cultural and demographic aspects of relative marriage in Iran. MA thesis in Demography, Faculty of Social Sciences, University of Tehran, Tehran

Tsuya NO, Mason KO (1995) Changing gender roles and below-replacement fertility in Japan. In: Mason KO, Jensen AM (eds) Gender and family change in industrialized countries. Clarendon Press, Oxford, pp 138–167

Chapter 9
Women's Autonomy and Fertility Behaviour

Introduction

Autonomy defined as 'the capacity to manipulate one's personal environment' indicates the technical, social, and psychological ability to obtain information and to use it in decision making processes regarding one's private concerns and those of one's intimates' (Dyson and Moore 1983, p. 45). The concept of autonomy is multi-dimensional, and includes information autonomy, decision-making autonomy, physical autonomy, emotional autonomy, and economic autonomy (Mason 1984; Mahadevan et al. 1989; Jejeebhoy 1996). Some studies have dealt with women's autonomy as an individual characteristic, while others have extended the scope of autonomy to include the capacity to act in the public realms of the labour market and social structure beyond one's household (Jejeebhoy 1996; Smith 1989; Morgan et al. 2002).

It has been argued that women's autonomy has considerable impact on reproductive behaviour. Women with higher autonomy are more likely to be involved in their marriage arrangements leading to a later age at marriage, to acquire information regarding family planning methods and to use the methods during their reproductive life, and to control their fertility (Jejeebhoy 1996). McDonald (2000) postulates that the fall from high to moderate levels of fertility is associated with fundamental improvements in women's autonomy within the family setting. Evidence on the relationship between women's autonomy and fertility and the degree to which these two variables are interrelated is mixed.

Support has been found for a relationship between women's autonomy and reproductive behaviour (Sathar et al. 2001; Hakim et al. 2003), but Morgan et al. (2002) concluded that the impact of women's autonomy on fertility in Muslim- and non-Muslim settings in different countries of Southeast Asia was not significant. It may be argued that the socio-cultural context of each setting can have considerable impact on women's autonomy and the extent to which it can affect fertility. For instance, Sankar Saikia et al. (2001, p. 16) noted that 'in an environment with pro-natalist social and cultural norms and a strong traditional society, high female autonomy may encourage women to produce more children'. Makhlouf Obermeyer (1994, p. 50) argued that gender equity and autonomy depend upon the socio-political context of the society in which the gender equity is discussed.

M.J. Abbasi-Shavazi et al., *The Fertility Transition in Iran: Revolution and Reproduction*,

Women's Status in Pre-and Post-revolutionary Iran

During the twentieth century, Iran has witnessed several policies and programs to improve the status of women. In the 1920s, Reza Pahlavi enacted laws that increased the minimum age at marriage to 14 years for girls, passed a compulsory education act, and tried to force women to abandon the veil. During the 1960s and 1970s, several steps were taken to improve the status of women as a component of the population policy. Work opportunities for women were increased as a result of which women's employment increased to around 14% by 1976. The legal minimum age at marriage for women was increased to 15. In 1975, the Family Protection Law limited the unilateral right of men to divorce as well as the practice of polygamy without the consent of the first wife. These movements were not implemented fully, but their symbolic values were very important, indicating that women's rights were officially recognized (Hoodfar 1995; Makhlouf Obermeyer 1994). However, as these policies ran counter to the more conservative cultural and religious values in the society, they were rejected by the opposition as Western-oriented and un-Islamic.

Soon after the revolution, the Islamic government emphasized domesticity and motherhood as the main roles of women, and reversed some of the policies initiated during the Shah's regime. For example, the legal minimum ages at marriage for boys and girls were reduced to 15 and 12, respectively. Wearing of the *Hijab* (veil) was made compulsory (Moghadam 2003). Primary, secondary and high schools were segregated for boys and girls. The presence of women in offices was discouraged, and thus, employment opportunities for women became more restricted. The Family Protection Law became ineffective and men were given unilateral rights for divorce as well as the practice of polygamy.

On the other hand, education for women was encouraged after the revolution. Rural families in particular were motivated to send their daughters to school. As a consequence, the education levels rose rapidly especially for women. Children of all social classes, including the poor, had access to education. Iranian girls now stay more years in school and university and, for many, this has delayed marriage and childbearing into the early 20s. The sex ratio of university students moved strongly in favour of girls. In 1998, around 52% of university candidates who were admitted to government universities were girls. The figure increased to 57% in 1999 and then to around 62% in 2001 (Abdollahyan 2004). Hoodfar (1996, p. 35) noted that increased literacy has contributed to women's confidence and has increased women's perceptions that they have options in many aspects of their lives. This was particularly the case for rural women whose opportunities had been highly constrained by traditional social norms. However, the substantial change in women's education in Iran was not translated into an increased level of paid employment for women in Iran, as women's employment remained below 15% in 2000.

The status of the wife within the couple relationship is also affected by the age difference between the husband and the wife. The difference in the mean ages at marriage of men and women in Iran has fallen from 6.6 years in 1966 to 3.1 years in 2006, although most of this fall occurred before 1986. This reduction in the age difference would have led to higher levels of communication between husbands and wives.

In many ways, the Islamic revolution has defined women's lives much more precisely than had previously been the case. Certain activities are permitted while others are not permitted. Women can be highly educated and can move around relatively freely, they can participate in women's groups especially religious and political groups and their education commands a higher level of respect from their husbands. At the same time, they must strictly observe the Islamic dress code, access to paid employment is very limited and, ultimately, they are under the authority of their husbands. Education for women is a pathway to refinement and respect, not for employment. For urban middle class women, this has represented a loss of freedom compared to the pre-1980 period while, for rural women, it has constituted an increase in freedom. With a relatively high degree of success, the Islamic revolution has attempted to converge Iranian women to an idealised type, at least in their public image. Individuality is not encouraged. This is much less the case for men and, in this regard, levels of gender equity in Iran are low. On the other hand, there is little question that education has provided rural women with more respect and decision-making power within the family, greatly increasing their levels of gender equity.

Despite these changes in the lives of Iranian women, few studies have been undertaken to examine the relationship between women's autonomy and fertility, and the extent to which women's autonomy can explain observed fertility differentials. This chapter will explore the level of women's autonomy, and the extent to which it has contributed to fertility differences in the four provinces included in the 2002 Iran Fertility Transition Survey. The objectives of the study are, first, to measure various dimensions of women's autonomy and investigate whether the selected provinces under scrutiny vary in terms of women's autonomy; and second, to analyse the relationship between women's autonomy and the use of contraception and ideal fertility.

Data and Setting

The 2000 Iran Fertility Transition Survey questionnaire included around 100 questions on various demographic and socio-economic characteristics as well as attitudes of women to children, marriage, women's employment and gender equity within and outside the family. The IFTS also adopted several questions from the study of women's autonomy in five Asian countries (Sathar et al. 2001) to operationalise the concept of women's autonomy, and to examine its relationship with reproductive behaviour. In addition to questions about education, work status as well as other attitudes regarding children, women were asked about various dimensions of autonomy including their decision-making authority, their freedom of movement, control over economic resources, and being afraid of their husbands or if they were ever beaten by their husbands.

The IFTS provides an excellent opportunity to examine women's autonomy in the four selected provinces of Sistan and Baluchistan, West Azarbaijan, Gilan and

Yazd with different demographic, socio-economic and cultural backgrounds. First, these provinces have displayed very different fertility levels and trends (Chapter 3). Second, there are substantial ethnic variations between the selected provinces. For example, Sistan and Baluchistan is populated mainly by *Baluchi*, while West Azarbaijan contains two large ethnic groups namely *Turks* and *Kurds*. The people living in the two other provinces are mainly *Persians*. Furthermore, a considerable proportion of the population in both Sistan and Baluchistan and West Azarbaijan are Sunni Muslims while the population in Yazd and Gilan are predominantly Shiite. Third, socio-economic characteristics such as literacy, employment, and access to electricity and safe water vary markedly across these provinces. Sistan and Baluchistan stands out with the lowest level of socio-economic development while Gilan and Yazd approach the highest levels of socio-economic development in the country. Selected development characteristics are illustrated in Table 9.1.

Women in Yazd enjoyed high levels of home and car ownership. Their access to modern goods in the household was considerably higher than in other provinces. Women in urban areas were better off in terms of car ownership and access to modern goods than their rural counterparts. Women in Gilan and Yazd had higher levels of education than women in the other two provinces. For example, around 60% of women in Sistan and Baluchistan and 48% of women in West Azarbaijan were illiterate as compared with 26% and 16% of women in Gilan and Yazd, respectively. With recent improvement in education, these provincial differences would be less pronounced at younger ages.

Women in Gilan and Yazd were also more likely to be employed than those in the other two provinces. In Gilan, women are employed in agriculture and, in Yazd, they are employed in carpet weaving. As expected, women in these two provinces

Table 9.1 Developmental characteristics by province and area of residence, 2002 IFTS

	Province				Area		
Index	Gilan	West Azarbaijan	Sistan and Baluchistan	Yazd	Rural	Urban	Total
Household indicator %							
Home ownership	71.6	74.2	76.6	81.2	78.1	71.5	74.6
Car ownership	20.0	27.0	18.2	41.4	17.3	31.1	24.5
Having four modern household goods[a]	17.3	17.6	11.1	52.3	3.8	35.3	20.3
Women's education level %							
Illiterate	26.0	48.0	59.3	15.9	53.0	25.9	38.9
Primary	28.1	25.9	21.9	48.7	28.9	28.2	28.5
Secondary	24.8	17.3	10.7	14.8	13.4	22.8	18.3
Diploma +	21.1	8.8	8.1	20.6	4.7	23.1	14.3
Women's economic independency %							
Employed	46.2	24.8	9.3	34.8	39.1	22.5	30.4
Have a private income	34.5	22.0	12.0	25.8	28.5	21.4	24.8
No. of women	1,222	1,317	1239	1,209	2,531	256	4,987

[a] The items included are colour TV, telephone, vacuum cleaner and washing machine.

were more likely to have a private income. Reflecting the industries of employment, women in rural areas were more likely than women in urban areas to be employed and to have access to a private income.

Our general observations suggest that these provinces also vary in terms of attitudes towards women. In Yazd, women's mobility outside the home as well as their social participation is controlled by conservative values, while more liberal views on women's mobility apply in Gilan. Both ethnicity and culture have influenced the position of women in the two provinces of West Azarbaijan and Sistan and Baluchistan. In West Azarbaijan, *Kurds* and *Turks* have different values toward women, although both ethnic groups are patriarchal in nature. In Sistan and Baluchistan, the Baluchi follow the Sunni sect of Islam and have their own particular culture.

Women's autonomy can be considered as an aggregate level or individual level factor. For example, following the strategy suggested by Smith (1989); Morgan et al. (2002) adopted a comparative research design that featured variation at the macro level. Their analysis included 14 community comparisons, focusing primarily on pairwise differences in community means with regards to measures of women's autonomy and fertility. At the aggregate level, if the four provinces in this study are arrayed from highest to lowest autonomy, the order would be Gilan, Yazd, West Azarbaijan and Sistan and Baluchistan. Fertility levels in these provinces were, respectively, 1.9, 2.3, 2.2 and 3.5 (Table 9.2). Thus, there is a relationship between women's autonomy and fertility at the aggregate level. However, this relates to only four provinces and if we divide the sample by urban and rural areas, the sample increases only to eight. This may not be large enough to draw a reliable conclusion. Therefore, the analysis in the chapter focuses upon the association of women's autonomy with ideal family size and use of contraception at the individual level. It is hypothesized that provinces with higher women's autonomy will have lower ideal fertility than those with lower women's autonomy. In particular, it is expected that women in Gilan and Yazd provinces enjoy higher autonomy than those in Sistan Baluchistan and West Azarbaijan provinces. Controlling for other demographic and development variables, we expect an inverse relationship between women's autonomy and low ideal fertility in the four provinces. Second, we expect lower contraceptive use among women with lower autonomy.

Table 9.2 Reproductive indicators by province, area and religion, 2002 IFTS

	Province				Area		
Index	Gilan	West Azarbaijan	Sistan and Baluchistan	Yazd	Rural	Urban	Total
Mean ideal fertility	1.9	2.2	3.5	2.3	2.6	2.1	2.4
Contraceptive use %							
All methods	79.2	79.4	46.5	80.1	67.8	77.6	72.9
Sterilization methods	19.1	21.8	7.3	23.9	18	18.5	18.2
Other modern methods	32.5	46.7	35	34.6	39.6	36.6	38.1
Traditional methods	27.6	10.9	4.2	21.6	10.2	22.5	16.6
No method	20.8	20.6	53.5	19.9	32.2	22.4	27.1

Several indices of female autonomy are used measuring such dimensions as mobility, decision-making, access and control over resources and freedom from threat or from ever being beaten by husband.

Fertility Differences

Table 9.2 shows the provincial variation in the dependent variables, ideal fertility and contraceptive usage. Mean ideal fertility is lowest in Gilan at a below replacement level of 1.9 births. The ideal is just above replacement in West Azarbaijan and Yazd but well above three births in Sistan and Baluchistan. Contraceptive prevalence rates (all methods) were very high in the three provinces of Gilan, West Azarbaijan and Yazd (around 80%) while the figure was around 47% in Sistan and Baluchistan. The use of traditional as well as sterilization methods was high among women in Yazd and Gilan provinces.

Differences in Women's Autonomy

The provincial differences in the explanatory variables (women's autonomy) are shown in Table 9.3. In general, the results indicate that women in Gilan and Yazd provinces experienced higher levels of autonomy in terms of economic decision-making, mobility, freedom from threat, and access to and control over resources as compared with women in West Azarbaijan and Sistan and Baluchistan. The level of women's autonomy in liberal Gilan was higher than in conservative Yazd province. Women in West Azarbaijan were more likely to be afraid of their husbands or to have ever been beaten by their husbands. Interestingly, despite its low levels of education and development, women in Sistan and Baluchistan were less likely to have been beaten by their husbands than was the case in the other provinces. As previously discussed, the Baluch have very high levels of consanguinity and this

Table 9.3 Measures of individual autonomy for women by province and area, 2002 IFTS

	Province				Area		
Index	Gilan	West Azarbaijan	Sistan and Baluchistan	Yazd	Rural	Urban	Total
Has no share in buying household items	3.9	11.5	23.6	5.2	14.0	7.4	10.5
Has no option to buy a present for others from the family's income	19.0	47.6	40.5	38.9	39.1	31.8	35.3
Has no option to transfer or sell property to others	34.4	63.3	41.8	53.1	54.0	42.2	47.8
Afraid of husband	29.6	71.4	63.1	43.0	58.4	46.1	52.0
Ever beaten by husband	36.8	51.1	29.6	34.7	43.0	37.2	39.9
Can go nowhere alone	9.5	31.1	62.6	16.4	34.2	22.6	28.1

may restrict domestic violence to some extent. Women in urban areas had more autonomy than their counterparts in rural areas. Women in Gilan had the highest freedom of mobility and women in Sistan and Baluchistan the lowest.

Women's Autonomy and Reproductive Indicators: Bivariate Associations

Table 9.4 shows the bivariate associations of various measures of women's autonomy and economic status with ideal fertility. The mean score of autonomy and economic status indices (scaled 0–10) is shown for each category of the dependent variable by province. The first five variables in the table are measures of the autonomy of women. These are followed by two measures of economic status. The final two columns in Table 9.4 are summary measures cumulated respectively from the five autonomy variables and the two economic status variables. The measures are explained in detail in Appendix. The dependent variable (ideal fertility) is divided into two categories of one to two or three and more children.

When the five indicators of women's autonomy are considered, in general, women with low ideal family sizes had higher autonomy scores. Likewise, those with low fertility ideals had higher scores on the two economic status measures. Accordingly, when the two summary measures of autonomy and economic status were considered, women with the lower fertility ideal had more autonomy and higher economic status than those with higher fertility ideals.

Table 9.4 Mean score of autonomy and economic status indices (scaled 0–10) by number of ideal children and province, 2002 IFTS

Region	No. of ideal children	Economic decision making	Freedom from threat	Mobility freedom	Access to economic resources	Control over economic resources	Modern goods ownership	Property ownership	Women's autonomy	Economic status
Sistan and Baluchistan	3+	4.35	6.02	1.81	5.02	1.96	1.67	3.27	3.70	3.58
	1–2	5.24	5.76	3.22	6.05	2.86	3.16	3.50	4.62	4.16
West Azarbaijan	3+	4.85	3.60	3.31	4.81	1.62	3.41	4.17	3.71	4.23
	1–2	4.96	4.38	3.94	5.64	2.02	4.24	4.30	4.27	4.77
Yazd	3+	5.16	5.71	5.52	6.16	2.12	4.85	5.57	4.84	5.44
	1–2	5.51	6.47	5.31	6.66	2.36	5.63	5.26	5.16	5.83
Gilan	3+	5.25	4.84	5.95	6.94	3.47	3.17	4.21	5.41	4.33
	1–2	5.47	6.71	6.77	7.04	3.57	4.19	4.10	5.81	4.89

Table 9.5 Mean score of autonomy and economic status indices (scaled 0–10) by contraceptive use and province, 2002 IFTS

Region	Method	Economic decision making	Freedom from threat	Mobility freedom	Access to economic resources	Control over economic resources	Modern goods ownership	Property ownership	Women's autonomy	Economic status
Sistan and Baluchistan	None	4.3	5.8	1.7	5.0	2.1	1.5	3.1	3.7	3.5
	Modern	5.1	6.0	3.0	5.9	2.5	3.0	3.7	4.4	4.0
	Traditional	6.0	7.2	5.0	7.2	3.8	5.1	4.3	5.8	5.6
West Azarbaijan	None	5.0	4.3	3.5	5.1	1.7	3.8	4.0	3.9	4.6
	Modern	4.9	4.0	3.8	5.4	1.9	3.9	4.2	4.1	4.5
	Traditional	5.2	5.2	4.5	6.6	2.5	5.5	5.0	4.9	5.7
Yazd	None	5.4	6.3	5.3	6.4	2.3	5.0	4.7	5.0	5.5
	Modern	5.4	6.1	5.4	6.5	2.3	5.4	5.5	5.0	5.7
	Traditional	5.5	6.7	5.4	6.7	2.1	5.8	5.5	5.2	5.9
Gilan	None	5.3	6.0	6.4	6.9	3.7	4.0	4.1	5.6	4.8
	Modern	5.6	6.4	6.7	6.9	3.4	3.8	4.1	5.7	4.7
	Traditional	5.4	7.3	7.0	7.4	3.7	4.8	4.1	6.0	5.2

In a similar form, Table 9.5 shows the bivariate association of contraceptive usage with the measures of autonomy and economic status. The dependent variable is divided into the three categories of modern method users, traditional method users, and non-users. Overall, with some exceptions, when the five measures of women's autonomy were considered, those who used modern and traditional methods were more autonomous than non-users. Consistent with the already observed associations of use of traditional methods by urban educated women, autonomy scores for women that used traditional methods were higher than for those that used modern methods. Again with some exceptions, the same general pattern applied to the two economic status measures; non-users had lower economic status than users and modern method users had lower scores than traditional method users. The general pattern holds when the two summary measures of autonomy and economic status are used although the differences between the mean scores for the three categories were relatively small in most cases.

Women's Autonomy and Ideal Family Size: Multivariate Associations

We now turn to a set of multivariate results that provide clues of possible causal relationships. Odds ratios in the Table 9.6 are estimated using logistic regression. Ideal fertility at the survey (low ideal fertility = one to two children vs. high ideal fertility = three or more children) is the dependent variable. Independent variables used in this analysis are education, province, the summary measure of economic

Table 9.6 Logistic Regression analysis predicting probability (odds ratio) of having a low ideal fertility (ideal fertility of one to two children) in four selected provinces of Iran, 2002 IFTS

Predictors	Model 1		Model 2		Model 3		Model 4	
Mobility:								
Can go nowhere alone (ref.)								
Can go some or all places alone			**	1.37	**	1.34		
Afraid of or beaten by husband: Either fearing or beaten or both (ref.)								
Neither fearing nor beaten					ns	1.08		
Having option to sell or transfer her properties to others:								
No option (ref.)								
Full or somewhat					*	1.17		
Having option to buy a present for others:								
No option (ref.)								
Full or somewhat					ns	1.09		
Autonomy: scaled 0–10							**	1.16
Household economic status:	*	1.05	ns	1.05	ns	1.04	ns	1.03
Scaled 0–10								
Education level:								
Illiterate (ref.)								
Primary	**	1.99	**	1.92	**	1.88	**	1.82
Secondary	**	3.39	**	3.19	**	3.08	**	2.98
Diploma+	**	5.45	**	5.04	**	4.69	**	4.20
Age group:								
<30 (ref.)								
30–39	ns	0.93	ns	0.91	ns	0.90	ns	0.87
40+	ns	0.89	ns	0.84	ns	0.83	*	0.80
Province:								
Sistan and Baluchistan (ref.)								
West Azarbaijan	**	4.87	**	4.53	**	4.89	**	5.22
Yazd	**	2.02	**	1.81	**	1.93	**	2.00
Gilan	**	11.41	**	10.02	**	10.08	**	9.89
Constant	**	0.44	**	0.41	**	0.36	**	0.28
Number included in the model		4,705		4,677		4,660		4,611

ns, not significant at 0.5 level.
* Significant at 0.5 level; ** significant at 0.01 level.

status and the set of women's autonomy measures used in the bivariate analysis. Four models are presented. Model 1 excludes all the women's autonomy measures but includes all the other explanatory variables. Model 2 adds in one of the autonomy measures, the mobility measure. Model 3 includes all four measures of women's autonomy. Finally, Model 4 replaces the four autonomy measures used in Model 3 with the summary measure of autonomy.

Model 1 shows that, controlling for other factors in the model, women in Gilan were 11 times more likely to have low ideal fertility (one to two children) than those from Sistan and Baluchistan. Women in West Azarbaijan and Yazd were five times and twice as likely respectively to have a low ideal fertility than women in Sistan and Baluchistan. Once education and economic status are controlled, women in Yazd were more similar to the reference group than women in the other two provinces. As expressed before, Yazd remains conservative in its ideals although its fertility behaviour has changed. The effect of education is also very significant and in the expected direction. Those with a diploma or higher education were around five times more likely to have a low fertility ideal than illiterate women. The effect of the summary measure of economic status is significant but small. After controlling for other factors, age is not significant.

Model 2 adds the effect of the mobility measure of autonomy. This was added as preliminary analysis indicated that it had the highest effect among the four measures of women's autonomy. It is highly significant with those having some freedom being 37% more likely to have a low fertility ideal than those with no freedom.

The third model in Table 9.6 includes all measures of autonomy. The effects of province and education remain very strong and significant when all four autonomy measures are included. Among the autonomy measures, the mobility measure (<0.01) and control over resources (<0.05) were significantly associated with low ideal fertility. The effects of the other three autonomy measures were not significant.

Finally, in Model 4, the summary measure of autonomy is substituted for the four autonomy measures in Model 3. The summary measure is significant but its effect is relatively small, even smaller than the effect of the single measure of mobility. Overall, the results suggest that women's autonomy has a significant effect on fertility ideals but the effect is very small compared with the effects of province and education.

Women's Autonomy and Contraceptive Usage: Multivariate Associations

The same analysis is undertaken for the relationship between women's autonomy and current contraceptive use (Table 9.7). Current contraceptive use is the dependent variable (yes vs. no). The independent variables used in this analysis are the same as those in Table 9.6 and the models are the same.

From Model 1, the province of residence again has highly significant effects although, in this case, the main differences are between Sistan and Baluchistan and the other three provinces. The size of the effect is similar for Yazd, West Azarbaijan and Gilan. Interestingly, once age, education and economic status are controlled, usage is higher in West Azarbaijan than in the other provinces. Education is also significant but, again, the differences between the effects for secondary education and higher education are small. Indeed, those with secondary education are a little more likely to be users than those with higher education. Usage is not affected by economic status. Thus, excluding Sistan and Baluchistan, usage of contraception was so common in these provinces that the conventional explanatory variables such as education had little effect. With lower levels of education than Yazd (Table 9.1),

Table 9.7 Logistic Regression analysis predicting probability (odds ratio) of using contraception to avoid pregnancy in four selected provinces of Iran, 2002 IFTS

Predictors		Model 1		Model 2		Model 3		Model 4
Mobility:								
Can go nowhere alone (ref.)								
Can go some/all where alone			**	1.57	**	1.57		
Afraid of or beaten by husband:								
Either fearing or beaten or both (ref.)								
Neither fearing nor beaten					ns	0.98		
Having option to sell or transfer her properties to others:								
No option (ref.)								
Full or somewhat					ns	1.05		
Having option to buy a present for others:								
No option (ref.)								
Full or somewhat					ns	0.99		
Autonomy: scaled 0–10							**	1.10
Household economic status: scaled 0–10	ns	1.02	ns	1.01	ns	1.02	ns	1.00
Education level:								
Illiterate (ref.)								
Primary	**	1.87	**	1.79	**	1.79	**	1.81
Secondary	**	2.52	**	2.32	**	2.32	**	2.36
Diploma+	**	2.33	**	2.14	**	2.13	**	2.06
Age group:								
<30 (ref.)								
30–39	**	2.17	**	2.10	**	2.08	**	2.10
40+	*	1.20	ns	1.11	ns	1.11	ns	1.15
Province:								
Sistan and Baluchistan (ref.)								
West Azarbaijan	**	3.94	**	3.51	**	3.56	**	4.00
Yazd	**	3.31	**	2.82	**	2.81	**	3.18
Gilan	**	3.19	**	2.63	**	2.63	**	2.83
Constant	**	0.47	**	0.44	**	0.42	**	0.36
Number included in the model		4,708		4,680		4,663		4,614

ns, Not significant at 0.5 level.
* Significant at 0.5 level; ** significant at 0.01 level.

West Azarbaijan is able to attain a similar level of usage (Table 9.2). This is confirmed by these multivariate results. As a control variable, the effect of age is significant and is as expected with highest usage being among women in their 30s.

In Model 2, the effect of the mobility measure of autonomy on contraceptive usage is significant and relatively large; those with some mobility are 57% more likely to be users than those with no mobility. The inclusion of this autonomy measure lowers the size of the both the education effects and the provincial effects. In Model 3, with the introduction of all four autonomy measures, the effects of all of the measures used in Model 2 remain the same as in Model 2 and none of the other three autonomy measures is significant. Finally in Model 4, the summary measure of autonomy is significant but the size of the effect is much smaller than the single mobility measure of autonomy. As women have to leave their households in order to access contraception, it is not unexpected that those that have no mobility are constrained in accessing supply points. As mobility is lowest in Sistan and Baluchistan, in Model 1, the effect of mobility becomes absorbed into the province measure. Likewise, some of the effect of mobility is absorbed into education in Model 1 because lack of mobility is associated with lower levels of education.

Summary and Discussion

Household and development indicators varied considerably across provinces. Women in Yazd and Gilan were better off than women in West Azarbaijan and Sistan and Baluchistan. Also, women in Gilan and Yazd provinces experienced higher levels of autonomy across all measures of autonomy (economic decision-making, mobility, freedom from threat, and access to and control over resources) compared with women in West Azarbaijan and Sistan and Baluchistan.

The findings indicate a significant, association between women's autonomy and reproductive behaviour. However, the pre-eminent aspect of autonomy in this regard was found to be freedom of mobility. When other socio-economic and demographic characteristics were controlled, those with some freedom of mobility were 37% more likely to have a low ideal family size and 57% more likely to be a user of contraception. At the same time, province and education were found to be the most important variables predicting ideal fertility and contraceptive use indicating the importance of the socio-cultural context of the four provinces for reproductive behaviour (see also Ali-Mondegari 2005). Once other variables were controlled, household economic status had no impact on ideal family size or upon use of contraception.

Makhlouf Obermeyer (1992, p. 50) argued socio-cultural factors are important determinants of both autonomy and reproductive behaviour and the findings here are consistent with this view. Cultural variables as summarised in the 'province' variable, were most important in shaping attitudes and behaviours on women's autonomy. This was confirmed by the fact that women in Yazd, despite enjoying higher levels of education and development, had slightly lower autonomy than women in Gilan reflecting the different cultures and values (conservative versus liberal) relating to women in these two provinces. On the other hand, although women in Sistan and Baluchistan had the lowest levels of education and development, they were much less likely to be afraid or beaten by their husbands as compared to women in West Azarbaijan. One measure of culture, the ability for women to move freely to places where they need to go, clearly reduced the effects of province and therefore can be considered to be one of the cultural variables that vary across provinces. However, other measures of women's autonomy considered in this analysis had no further impact in reducing the effects of province. Further research is required to examine what other cultural variables that vary across provinces may have an impact on reproductive health. It may not be possible to isolate these variables in quantitative terms.

In summary, women's autonomy, especially their capacity to move freely, has a clear impact on reproductive health outcomes in Iran. However, the effects of education and province (unmeasured cultural variables) are much stronger. These effects, however, cannot be considered to be independent of each other as education increases women's autonomy at the individual level. This is consistent with the argument made by Kasarda et al. (1986, p. 87) who considered 'education as an engine of status enhancement'.

Appendix: 9.1

Dependent Variables

1. Contraceptive use: Women were asked whether they were currently using any kind of contraceptive method to avoid pregnancy. Contraceptive use was considered as a dichotomous variable and coded as 0 if women were not currently using any method and 1 if currently using a contraceptive method. There are no missing values for this variable and 1,423 (27.1%) women were not using any contraceptive and 3,564 (72.9%) were using a contraceptive method.
2. Ideal fertility: Women are divided into two categories to make a dichotomous variable and coded as 0 if women had low ideal fertility (one to two children) and 1 if they had high ideal fertility (three or more children).

Independent Variables

Demographic characteristics of women: There were no missing values for any of the demographic variables that include:

Province: A nominal variable with four categories with roughly equal numbers.

Age: An interval variable that is categorized into three groups: 0 = <30, 1 = 30–39, and 2 = 40+.

Educational status: Originally an ordinal variable with ten categories from illiterate to university level. It was grouped into four categories: illiterate, primary, secondary, and diploma or higher.

Economic status of the household:

Property ownership: An interval variable scaled from 0 to 6. It is a simple sum of the ownership of six types of property with values of 0 (ownership) and 1 (non-ownership). The types of property were: house; land, garden or factory; car; motorcycle; gold, jewels or silver; and saving accounts. There were 22 (0.4%) missing cases for this variable.

Modern goods ownership: An interval variable scaled from 0 to 8. It is a simple sum of the ownership of eight modern durables with values of 0 (ownership) and 1 (non-ownership). The types of goods were freezer, tape recorder, colour TV, video, telephone, vacuum cleaner, washing machine and furniture. There were 13 (0.3%) missing cases for this variable.

Economic status index: This is a summary measure constructed by applying Principal Components Analysis taking into account the property, modern goods and per capita monthly expenditure of households. The following are the results and procedures of analysis:

One component out of three was above 1 and it explained 61.2% of the variance of the initial three variables.

The constructed component was correlated with the three initial variables.

The component was scaled from 0 to 10 (lowest economic status to highest economic status).

Women's autonomy

Economic decision-making: An interval variable scaled from 0 to 6. There were 9 (0.2%) missing cases for this variable. It is a simple sum of the role of women in making decisions on buying "Foodstuffs", "Household items" and "Gold and jewels" with values of 0 (no role), 1 (cooperative role) and 2 (independent role).

Access to economic resources: An interval variable scaled from 0 to 6. There are 53 (1.1%) missing cases for this variable. It is a simple sum of the responses of women to the following questions with values of 0 (no) and 1 (yes).

- Can you provide your ideas about how the family income is spent?
- Are you given any cash to spend?
- Do you have the option to buy presents for others?
- Do you have the option to buy a piece of gold for yourself?
- Do you have any source of income?
- Do you have any financial support or saving for your old age?

Control over economic resources: An interval variable scaled from 0 to 4. There were 42 (0.8%) missing cases for this variable. It is a simple sum of the responses of women to the following questions with values of 0 (no), 1 (partly) and 2 (totally).

- Do you have permission to sell or transfer your belongings to other people?
- Do you have any source of income and control over it?

Freedom from threat: An interval variable scaled from 0 to 3. There were eight (0.2%) missing cases for this variable. It is derived from two questions on whether women are afraid of or are ever beaten by their husbands and has the following values of 0 (not afraid of and not beaten by husband), 1 (afraid, but not beaten by husband), 2 (not afraid, but beaten by husband) and 3 (both afraid of and beaten by husband).

Freedom of mobility: An interval variable scaled from 0 to 15. There were 60 (1.2%) missing cases for this variable. It is calculated based on the mobility of women to the following places with values of 0 (must get permission of husband and be escorted by a family member), 1 (only must be escorted by a family's member), 2 (must get permission but can go alone) and 3 (can go alone without permission).

- Health clinic or doctor's office
- Religious ceremonies
- Relatives' homes

- Wedding ceremonies
- Neighbouring towns or villages

Autonomy index: This is a summary measure constructed by applying Principal Components Analysis taking into account decision-making, freedom of mobility, freedom from threat, access to economic resources and control over economic resources. The following are the results and procedures of analysis:

One component out of five was above 1 and it explained 54% of the variance of the initial three variables.

The constructed component was correlated with the five initial variables.

The component was scaled to 0–10 (no autonomy to high autonomy).

References

Abdollahyan H (2004) The generations gap in contemporary Iran. J Welt Trends 44:78–85

Alimondegari M (2005) Imapcts of various aspects of women's autonomy on fertility behaviours in Iran (Persian), MA Thesis, Department of Demography, University of Tehran, Tehran

Dyson T, Moore M (1983) On kinship structure, female autonomy, and demographic behavior in India. Popul Dev Rev 9(1):35–60

Hakim A, Salway S, Mumtaz Z (2003) Women's autonomy and uptake of contraception in Pakistan. Asia-Pacific Popul J 18(1):63–82

Hoodfar H (1995) Population policy and gender equity in post-revolutionary Iran. In: Makhlouf Obermeyer C (ed) Family, gender, and population in the Middle East. The American University in Cairo Press, Cairo, pp 105–135

Hoodfar H (1996) Bargaining with fundamentalism: women and the politics of population control in Iran. Reprod Health Matters 8:30–40

Jejeebhoy SJ (1996) Women's education, autonomy and reproductive behavior; assessing what we have learned. East West Center, Honolulu, HI

Kasarda JD, Billy JOC, West K (1986) Status enhancement and fertility: reproductive responses to social mobility and educational opportunity. Academic, Orlando, FL

Mahadevan K, Aghajanian A, Jayasree R, Moni GS (1989) Status of women and population dynamics: a conceptual model. In: Mahadevan K (ed) Women and population women dynamics: perspectives from Asian countries. Sage, New Delhi, pp 345–379

Makhlouf Obermeyer C (1994) Reproductive choice in Islam: gender and state in Iran and Tunisia. Stud Fam Plan 25(1):41–51

Mason K (1984) The status of women: a review of its relationship to fertility and mortality. Rockefeller Foundation, New York

McDonald P (2000) Gender equity in theories of fertility transition. Popul Dev Rev 26(30): 427–439

Moghadam VM (2003) Modernizing women: gender and social change in the Middle East, 2nd edn. Lynne Rienner, Boulder, CO

Morgan P, Smith H, Satar S, Mason KO (2002) Muslim and non-Muslilm differences in female autonomy and fertility. Popul Dev Rev 28(3):515–537

Sathar Z, Callum C, Jejeebhoy S (2001) Gender, region, region and reproductive behavior in India and Pakistan. Paper presented at the IUSSP conference, Salvador, Brazil, 12–14 Aug 2001

Sankar Saikia U, Steele R, Dasvarma G (2001) Culture, religion and reproductive behavior in two indigenous communities of northeastern India: a discussion of some preliminary findings. Paper presented at the IUSSP conference, Salvador, Brazil, 12–14 Aug 2001

Smith H (1989) Integrating theory and research on the institutional determinants of fertility. Demography 26:171–184

Chapter 10
Explanations of the Past and Expectations of the Future of Fertility in Iran

Introduction

In this book, we have set out to contribute to knowledge of the determinants of the fertility transition, the movement of a country's fertility rate from a high level to a moderate or low level. We are fortunate in that in the case that we use, Iran, the decline is recent and it has occurred over a short period of time. The recency of the decline has meant that we were able to collect new data in the 2002 and 2005 surveys from the women who were at the forefront of the fertility transition. We were able to examine their behaviour and their motivations in great detail. In particular, in the 2005 survey, we obtained a full, month by month history of the women's contraceptive usage histories that covered the full period of the fertility transition. And we were able to relate these contraceptive histories to the changes in fertility in Iran across time.

The recency of the Iranian transition also enables us to benefit from the prior theoretical and empirical research undertaken by many other scholars relating to other countries. There is no shortage of plausible theories to explain fertility transition and the main theories have been reviewed in Chapter 1. Here we repeat the main theories and provide a summary assessment of the applicability of each one to the Iran fertility transition.

1. *Demographic transition theory*: fertility transition is a component of industrialization and urbanization with change in family structure from extended to nuclear.

As demographic transition theory is a very generally stated theory, it can be expected that the evidence will be mixed and this is the case for Iran. Confirming the theory, fertility has fallen faster in urban areas than in rural areas and in more developed provinces than in less developed provinces. Fertility has remained highest in the least developed of the provinces, Sistan and Baluchistan. Urbanisation and rural to urban migration were prominent across the period of the transition as was a degree of industrialization. The extended family no longer has a strong hold on young couples once married. In question of the theory, the falls in fertility in rural areas have been more dramatic than in urban areas and the province with the lowest fertility, Gilan, has a largely agrarian economy. Furthermore, the differences in timing of the falls in urban and rural areas are very short. Also, as indicated in Chapter 8, much about family life has remained traditional, especially the practice of consanguinity. Overall, the ubiquity of the transition across the country in a relatively short time frame is counter to the expectation of gradual change inherent in demographic transition theory.

2. *Improvement in child survival*: sharp falls in infant and child mortality provide parents with the security that their children will survive to adulthood and there is therefore less need to have larger numbers of children in order to ensure the survival of at least a few of them.

The Islamic revolution led to the spread of a quality health care system across Iran and this substantially reduced the levels of infant and child mortality. Certainly, by 2000, couples could be assured that a child born was very likely indeed to be a child that grew to adulthood. A high level of child survival has to be a necessary condition of any fertility transition. There are no recorded cases of countries where fertility has fallen rapidly in the context of continuing high infant and child mortality. However, there are instances in which infant and child mortality has fallen but fertility remains high. In this sense, higher child survival is not an automatic or sufficient condition for fertility decline. While there had been early improvements in infant and child mortality and this would have provided parents with a sense of security that the few children that they had would survive, the speed of decline was so rapid that it could not have been explained simply by prior falls in child mortality.

3. *Demand theory*: Like any commodity, the demand for children falls when the costs exceed the benefits. Benefits fall as children are no longer needed for household production or to provide old age security. Costs increase with compulsory education and the social requirement to produce 'high quality' children. This includes wealth flows theory which postulates that the demand for children falls when the net flow of wealth changes direction from children to parents to parents to children.

Today, all Iranian children complete primary school and a high proportion complete secondary school. However, the costs to Iranian parents of achieving these educational ends are not high. On the other hand, there is no great evidence that having many children was a major economic asset to Iranian families prior to the fertility transition. Furthermore, there is little support for an argument that having fewer children freed up women to engage in paid employment (reduction of the opportunity cost) as paid employment remains uncommon for Iranian mothers. Thus, a simply stated demand theory is unlikely to have played a major role in the Iranian transition. More pertinent is the notion that Iranian couples began to invest in the 'quality' of a small number of children as distinct from a large number of children of 'lower quality'. When education becomes widespread, success of children in the education system emerges as a new motivation for parents. A successful child provides status and the potential for economic support in later life from sons or a good marriage for daughters. Given that family resources are normally shared across all children, this implies that parents will demand a small number of children so that they can invest more in each child. This is not a simple cost-benefit equation. It is a strategy to maximize status and, perhaps, economic returns from the costs inevitably incurred in having children.

4. *Rising economic aspirations*: High economic aspirations are generated by modernization, globalisation, popular media and changes in the opportunity structure generated primarily by education. Both for countries and for households, a large number of children is seen as an obstacle to achieve economic betterment.

We consider that this theoretical argument has considerable power in the Iranian case. There were strong expectations on the part of the broad base of Iranian people that the Islamic revolution would bring them considerable economic reward. They perceived that Iran was a wealthy country (because of oil revenue) but that the distribution of wealth was inequitable. We have observed that fertility began to fall in the mid-1980s when economic conditions were poor. The strength of the fertility decline in these years (1986–1989), as we have observed, was masked to some extent by a marriage boom at the end of the Iran–Iraq war. By 1989, at the time of the revival of the family planning programme, fertility in Gilan and Tehran had fallen to 3.7 and 3.8 births per woman respectively. For Iran as a whole, fertility fell from 7.0 in 1984 to 5.3 in 1989. Thus, it is clearly evident that marital fertility was falling solidly in almost all provinces before the revival of the family planning programme (Abbasi-Shavazi and McDonald 2005). The difficulties that Iran has faced since the revolution (the Iran–Iraq war, economic sanctions, fluctuations in oil revenues, and inefficient organization of industrial production) have ensured that the economic realities that couples have faced since the revolution have fallen well short of the high expectations that people have developed. While basic needs are met in Iran to a very large extent, economic aspirations extend well beyond basic needs. In Chapter 8, we have shown that economic motivations were very strong in people's statements about having a small number of children or in not having a large number. This is a very strongly held view across the country.

To the extent that social aspirations can be separated from economic aspirations, the study has found little evidence to support the theory that Iranian couples have reduced their number of children in order to seek enhanced social status. While it would be considered to be socially unacceptable in today's Iran to have a very large number of children, moderate numbers such as three and four would not be considered as socially unacceptable, but most people do not have these numbers. Social status in Iran is variously defined. In many parts of Iran, religious participation is a component of social status. For women in urban areas, not easily able to pursue working careers, status is sometimes indicated by participation in 'refined' activities including music and art and familiarity with English literature. The number of children is not a strong determinant of participation in these activities.

5. *Gender equity theory*: As the status of women rises through education and changes in cultural values, women will gain more control over their own fertility. In advanced East Asian settings where fertility fell dramatically, education levels for women rose and age at first marriage increased substantially. Single women conventionally had long periods of paid employment before marrying. This enabled them to have a more equitable position in the family once they had married. In particular, their husbands were responsive to the desire on the part of wives to control their childbearing. It has also been argued that this result can occur even without an increase in women's status outside the family so long as her status within the family improves.

Like low levels of infant and child mortality, we would argue that higher levels of gender equity within the couple relationship are a necessary condition of fertility transition, but not necessarily a sufficient condition. Fertility falls only when women gain control over their own fertility. The study has shown that withdrawal is relatively commonly used in some cultural contexts in Iran in order to control fertility. And this practice seems to have a long history especially among the urban middle class in Tehran. Indeed, it may have become an integral part of the sexual practice of these couples. The practice of withdrawal implies a cooperative relationship between husband and wife. The extension of female education across Iran has contributed to a higher status for wives within the couple relationship. In rural areas, fertility control has been achieved primarily through female methods of contraception. That the use of contraception and the provision of family planning services to women were supported by religious leaders is also significant. Finally, the analysis in Chapter 9 found that freedom of mobility for women was associated with lower ideal family size and with use of contraception.

The family planning programme in rural areas was directed towards women. Improvements in women's education, increases in age at marriage, falls in the age gap between husbands and wives and improved status of women in the revolution all contributed to a capacity for women to make use of the programme. This was done with the support of husbands feeling economic pressure.

6. *Institutional change*: Changes in institutions such as education, government, gender and family, culture and the economy move in directions that favour lower fertility. A potentially important institutional change is the creation of a government-backed family planning program.

The Iranian fertility tradition was accompanied literally by revolutionary institutional changes. In the early years of the Islamic revolution, pronatalism and the abandonment of the family planning program led to a temporary increase in fertility for the country as a whole. The increases were highest in the more remote and least developed provinces. In Sistan and Baluchistan, the total fertility rate approached ten births per woman in these years. In the central provinces and the city of Tehran, fertility continued to fall in the early 1980s and pre-revolution levels of contraceptive usage were maintained. Most importantly, however, the revolution led to two major institutional changes that were fundamental to future fertility decline:

universal education for women including adult literacy programs and the development of a national health system that provided access to basic health resources to all Iranians. These provided the foundation for the implementation of the national family planning program in 1989.

We do not argue that the family planning program itself provided the motivation for smaller family size, however, it most definitely allowed women to implement their desires to control the number of children that they had. Fertility would probably have fallen in the major urban areas without the family planning program but the evidence in this book shows that the program had a huge impact on fertility levels in rural areas. Contraceptive use in most rural areas was and still is dependent upon the national delivery system through the Ministry of Health. The family planning program would not have been the success that it was, however, without the prior extension of the national health system across the country and without the greater autonomy provided to women through the national education system. The strong support provided to the family planning program by religious leaders both at the national and the local levels was a further important element in its success. Another important institution in our story is the Ministry of Health and Medical Education. The Ministry officials who ran the family planning program provided a program that was flexible and responsive to local cultural preferences. While prevalence rates for contraception use are very high in most parts of the country, the method mix varies across cultures fairly considerably, and this has been an important explanation of the high prevalence rates.

Finally, as discussed in Chapter 2, the family planning program was the end result of a change in population policy in the mid-1980s. Iranian demographers and public health officials were prominent at the time in convincing the government and the religious leaders that very high population growth was not in the nation's economic interests and the poor economic conditions in the mid 1980s helped in the reception of this message. The change in population policy also provided broad social permission for couples to control their fertility even though the family planning programme was not yet in place.

While these institutional changes were necessary conditions for the speed of the fertility decline, the very speed of adoption of contraception when it was made available in 1990 is indicative of a pent-up demand for contraception. As argued above, we suggest that this pent-up demand was a result of the divergence between economic aspirations and economic reality in the 1980s.

7. *Diffusion and ideation*: Fertility falls because of the spread of the idea that small families are better than large families. It is the idea that is important, not any structural or institutional changes behind the idea. Small family size is simply a good idea that has found its time and place.

Fertility falls with diffusion of the idea that limitation of the number of children in a family will enhance the family's economic wellbeing and improve the opportunities for advancement of the fewer children that the family has. Also, to use contraception effectively, people must know where to get it and how to use it. Thus, diffusion is also a necessary element in fertility transition. By mobilizing various government organizations and the mass communication network, the family planning program succeeded in diffusing ideas throughout the entire country about the value of small families and about methods of family limitation. The creation of an accessible national health system in the 1980s made it possible, from 1990, for the revived family planning programme to have a rapid impact, especially in rural areas.

Furthermore, the official program introduced by the government in 1989 enjoyed the support of religious leaders. Local religious leaders promoted family planning through the mosques.

An unusual feature of the Iranian fertility transition was the emergence of a very long interval between the first and the second birth. Spacing of births was promoted by the government program but not very long spacing of births. Furthermore, long spacing is evident in urban areas where the effect of the government program was not as strong. The adoption of long intervals between births seems to have been a spontaneous response to relatively early first births and the economic difficulties that faced young couples.

These ideas were only diffused across society, however, because there had been institutional changes that enabled this to happen: the change in population policy, the development of the national health system and the improvements in literacy of women. The ideas were enthusiastically adopted also, we would argue, because of the economic conditions that people faced in the latter part of the 1980s. Finally, increased levels of gender equity within the family meant that these ideas could be discussed in women's groups and between husband and wife.

8. *Tempo effects*: Delay of the first birth through delay of marriage or use of contraception before the first birth and wider spacing between births accelerate the speed of fertility decline because births are pushed out into the future.

In advanced East Asian countries, fertility fell in the context of substantial increases in age at first marriage. Later marriage produced an immediate, tempo effect upon period fertility rates as births were pushed out into the future. This is not a feature of the early years of the Iranian fertility transition as delays in age at marriage were modest. In this regard, the Iranian transition was more like the transition in Indonesia where increases in age at marriage were also modest in the early years. Because of its relatively conservative Islamic orientation, there have been limits in Iran in the extent to which age at first marriage can rise. The cultural constraint that women should marry at a relatively early age combined with the expectation that couples should have their first birth as soon as possible within marriage meant that tempo effects deriving from delay of the first birth were initially small. However, since the mid 1990s, age at marriage has been rising more rapidly and, as we argue below, there are good reasons to believe that it will rise even more in the future. Also by the late 1990s, there was evidence of a new trend for the first birth to be delayed within marriage (Hosseini-Chavoshi et al. 2006; Hosseini-Chavoshi 2007). Thus, a tempo effect arising from delay of marriage and the first birth has been building up as the transition has progressed.

An earlier tempo effect, however, derives from the widespread adoption of a substantial interval between the first and the second birth that emerged very early in the transition and gained strength thereafter. This had followed a tempo effect working in the opposite direction when a post-war marriage boom initially slowed down the fertility transition in the late 1980s. The juxtaposition of these two tempo effects working in opposite directions would have pushed period fertility downwards in the 1990s at a faster rate than otherwise would have been the case.

Concluding Remark

This study has involved a decade of research on the Iran fertility transition. The two specific data collections undertaken as part of the study were designed to consider the various possible theoretical explanations of the transition. It is apparent from the discussion in this chapter that no one theory provides a sufficient explanation of the transition. Indeed, most of the theories have had some applicability. We would argue that there are certain necessary conditions for a fertility transition to occur. These include the achievement of low levels of infant and child mortality, institutional changes that provide access to contraception and access to economic opportunity at least for the next generation, diffusion of the idea that limiting the number of children in the family will enhance the family's economic wellbeing and improve the opportunities of each child, and the establishment of communication between husband and wife to a level that provides the wife with the opportunity to exercise control over her own fertility. All of these necessary conditions were met in Iran.

If these necessary conditions are in place, then government and community support for family planning especially through an efficient and accessible national family planning program will accelerate the speed of the transition as it certainly did in Iran. It also seems inevitable that any fertility transition will be associated with tempo effects that will force period fertility down more rapidly than otherwise. These tempo effects will be associated with delay of the first birth and wider spacing between the births.

Finally, while the initial stages of the transition may be associated with limitation of births that would have been considered 'excess' even in the context prior to transition, the fall of fertility to replacement level must be associated with strong motivations to limit the number of births to two, or three if the desired gender composition of the children has not been achieved. This motivation can be sold to people through family planning propaganda and this was done to some extent in Iran. The motivation may derive from the emergence of life alternatives for women, notably the opportunity to pursue a career outside the household. This does not seem to have been important in the case of Iran. We conclude that, first and foremost in Iran, this motivation has an economic basis, the failure of economic reality for most Iranian households to come close to matching their economic aspirations.

Very low fertility (period total fertility below 1.5 births per woman) occurs when a tempo effect is so strong that fertility falls temporarily to this level or when a preference emerges for a one-child family. Tehran City and two provinces in Iran,

Gilan and Mazandaran, had fertility rates below 1.5 in 2006, with Gilan being as low as 1.2. A number of other provinces were approaching very low fertility with levels of 1.6 or 1.7 births per woman. These include Markazi, Isfahan, East Azerbaijan, Hamadan, Semnan and Ghazvin. These are all majority Persian provinces in the developed north of Iran. There is little doubt that these very low period fertility rates are artificially low because of tempo effects, however, even in 2002, a substantial minority in Gilan province expressed a preference for one child. This gives rise to the question as to how much lower Iranian fertility will fall. This question is taken up in the final section of the book.

The Future

Will fertility in Iran rise again in the near future, will it level off at the current level, or will it decline further? In what follows, we argue that Iran will experience further fertility decline during the coming decade. Necessarily the speed of the decline will be slow compared to the past decades. We will also speculate about the possibility of rising fertility in the future.

Continuing Fertility Decline

Several reasons justify further fertility decline in Iran during the coming decade, 2010–2020. First, provincial as well as rural and urban differences in fertility are still evident in Iran and we can expect these differences to narrow. Indeed, with the single exception of Sistan and Baluchistan where fertility remained above three births per woman in 2006, the trend data suggest that fertility in all provinces of Iran will soon fall below 2.0. The cultural (religion and ethnicity) and socio-economic (education, level of economic development) and political factors that explain relatively higher fertility in Sistan and Baluchistan will remain pertinent and fertility may well remain above 3.0 in this province over the next decade. It is instructive to remember, however, that fertility in Sistan and Baluchistan in the early 1980s approached ten births per woman.

Second, the continued process of urbanisation is another reason that lower fertility can be expected in the future. In 2006, around 68% of the population were living in urban areas and it has been estimated that, by 2020, around 75% of the population will live in urban areas. Urbanization will increase aspirations of couples for a better life but they will face the higher costs of housing in urban areas. This will in turn modify the reproductive behaviour of women in favour of smaller families and fewer children. Further, as Chesnais (2000: 126) argued, the impact of globalization on social life in other countries should not be ignored. No specific country or region can be seen in isolation from other countries in the exchange of ideas and culture today. However, Iran is less open to such influences than many other countries.

Third, the level of education continues to increase. Children of all social classes, including the poor, have access to education, and the educational differences in the society will be reduced further in the future. The level of education of young women has increased over the last two decades and women are now more educated than men (Abdollahyan 2004). This has resulted in increased gender equity within the household in Iran and women have the major role in fertility decision-making. Although the level of female employment is still low, given the rising expectations of Iranian women (Shadi-Talab 2005), it is likely that women's labour force participation will increase in the future. This result, however, is contingent upon there being sufficient jobs to absorb the very large numbers of young people recently entering the labour market.

Fourth, age at marriage for women is increasing significantly as a result of the increases in women's education. There is also economic pressure on new couples to have a job and house before they marry and the opportunities to achieve this are reducing as the large cohorts enter the labour and housing markets in urban areas. This is likely to delay marriage even further. Attitudes towards marriage have also changed and even traditional families do not consider marriage as the only option for their children. There is also a sex imbalance in the marriage ages in Iran, that is, the number of women in the marriage ages is higher than the number of men. This is because the number of men in the older cohort who were born immediately before the revolution is much smaller than the number of women in the next younger cohort who are the babies of the early post-revolution baby boom. Brides will be much less in demand and hence a lower proportion may marry or they will marry men more their own age. Again, later marriage is a likely outcome.

Fifth, for men in particular, as the decade progresses, the very large, post-revolutionary birth cohort will experience a highly competitive labour market. This will mean that they will need to invest even more in job searching and the building of their own human capital through education and work experience (Salehi-Isfahani 2008; Salehi-Isfahani and Egel 2007). These young cohorts are already experiencing very high levels of unemployment. In the 2006 Census, the unemployment rate was 30.7% for males aged 15–19 and 20.5% for males aged 20–24. This now comes together with the impact of the global economic recession that has seen oil prices fall dramatically. It is difficult to envisage in these circumstances how many from the very large cohorts of young men will be able to attain incomes adequate for them to marry and have children. The difference between economic aspirations and economic reality will become even wider.

Sixth, the higher status of women in Iran will also tend to have a negative effect on fertility in the future. This is in line with the 'gender equity' argument made by McDonald (2000) and supports Dyson's (2002) hypothesis that one of the main factors of the fall of fertility in developing countries is that 'women become more like men'. Shadi-Talab (2005) has also noted that "Iranian girls gradually practice democracy within the family, and patriarchal power is slowly diminishing. Although, attitudinal change is a very slow process, the interaction between education and changes in norms and values is observable in the share of girls' participation at universities from the most deprived provinces and far from their home town."

Commenting on gender equality in Iran, Mir-Hosseini (2002: 95) observed that "no political tendency can ignore the new generation of women who have come of age during the life of the Islamic Republic and who are demanding equal opportunities and rights on all fronts. Women are now a force that must be reckoned with" (see also, Kian-Thiebaut 2002: 56–73). On the other hand, the competition for jobs among young people in Iran is and will continue to be very strong and it may well eventuate that societal forces move to limit women's capacity to compete so as to favour jobs for young men. The discriminatory structure of employment both horizontally (limited job opportunities) and vertically (obstacles to job promotion and lower wages for women) is a challenge facing women's economic participation in Iran.

Seventh, as Caldwell et al. (2000) have argued, the contributions of governments to population control in Asian countries have been very important. The very large, post-revolutionary baby boom has already started having children. Even with low fertility, this will lead to a considerable increase in the number of births compared to recent years. Because of this 'echo effect', the Iranian Government has indicated that it shall maintain the family planning program. Population and family planning is still being taught as a compulsory unit to all university students. Considerable effort is concentrated on the improvement of health, the expansion of reproductive health services, as well as the reduction of fertility in rural areas and the provinces with high fertility. These programs have not only affected the attitudes of childbearing women, but also have shaped the fertility attitudes and behaviour of the young generation. In a counter direction, as observed in Chapter 1, President Ahmadinejad has raised the issue of low fertility as an obstacle to Iran's advancement as a nation and has commented that Iran could accommodate double its present population size. This political debate will be ongoing in the coming decade but, as observed in other countries, once low fertility norms have been established, it is very difficult for governments to reverse them. Women who were interviewed in the Iran Fertility Transition Survey (Abbasi-Shavazi et al. 2003) indicated that they would not increase their fertility even if the government provided incentives to do so.

A desire for small family size is a widely held ideal among Iranian women. The ideal family size of Iranian women is concentrated on two children. The results of the 2002 Iran Fertility Transition Survey conducted in the four selected provinces of Gilan, West Azarbaijan, Yazd and Sistan-Baluchistan showed that the majority of women, on average, desired only two children. Surprisingly, in Gilan province, around 24% of women aged 20–29 and around 18% of women aged 40–49 indicated one child as their ideal number of children (Abbasi-Shavazi et al. 2003). We have argued in Chapter 4 that the widespread adoption and implementation of a two-child family norm is the essential story of fertility decline in Iran.

Eighth, the effectiveness of family planning methods is another factor supporting fertility decline. According to the Iran Demographic and Health Survey, the contraceptive prevalence rate was around 72% in 2000. There exists a small gap between the level of CPR in rural and urban areas. However, a significant proportion of pregnancies (around 33%) were still unintended. Of these, around 18% were unwanted and 15% were mistimed (Abbasi-Shavazi et al. 2004). With the continued improvement of the quality of family planning services, the level of unwanted pregnancies is likely to be reduced, and thus, fertility might be expected to decline further. Current patterns of behaviour mean that many Iranian women complete their fertility before age 30 at which ages, sterilisations are generally not available. This can mean an increased risk of having an unwanted pregnancy and abortion. However, where abortions are difficult to obtain and if sterilization is not accepted or widespread at younger ages, contraceptive failure or non use could remain high and the level of unwanted births may not fall as expected.

Ninth, the long-held cultural beliefs that women should marry early and that they should have the first baby soon after marriage no longer hold much force. Age at marriage has been rising strongly in recent times and, as argued above, can be expected to continue to rise. The Iran Low Fertility Survey showed that 40% of couples in Tehran City in 2005 began their marriages using contraception in order to delay the first birth.

Tenth, when most women want to have two children, a tempo effect can temporarily reduce the annual fertility rate below two. The emergence of below replacement fertility in many parts of Iran is no doubt associated with a tempo effect. The question then becomes: how long will this tempo effect last? There is little scope for further delay of the second birth but there is considerable scope for further delay of the first birth. Given the severe economic competition facing the large cohorts now aged between 15 and 24, there is a strong likelihood that first births will be delayed particularly in urban areas. This might be through increased age at marriage or through delay of the first birth within marriage. This would keep fertility below replacement level for the next decade or so and it is more than likely, over the next decade, Iran will enter the ranks of countries having a very low fertility rate.

References

Abbasi-Shavazi MJ, McDonald P (2005) National and provincial-level fertility trends in Iran: 1972–2000. Working Paper in Demography, No. 94. The Australian National University, Canberra

Abbasi-Shavazi MJ, McDonald P, Hosseini Chavoshi M (2003) Changes in family, fertility behavior and attitudes in Iran. Working Paper in Demography No. 88. The Australian National University, Canberra

Abbasi-Shavazi MJ, Hosseini-Chavoshi M, Delavar B, Aghajanian A, Mehryar A (2004) Unintended pregnancies in the Islamic Republic of Iran: levels and correlates. Asia-Pacific Popul J 19(1):27–38

Abdollahyan H (2004) The generations gap in contemporary Iran. J Welt Trends 44:78–85

Caldwell J, Caldwell P, McDonald P (2000) Consequences of low fertility and policy responses: a global perspective, in Korea Institute for Social Affairs and United Nations Population Fund, Low Fertility and Policy Responses to Issues of Ageing and Welfare, KIHASA, Seoul

Chesnais JC (2000) Determinants of below-replacement fertility. In: Below replacement fertility, Population Bulletin of the United Nations, New York, pp 126–136

Dyson T (2002) On the future of human fertility in India. Paper prepared for the Expert Group Meeting on Continuing the Fertility Transition. Population Division of the United Nations, New York, 11–14 March 2002

Hosseini-Chavoshi M (2007) Fertility regulation in Iran: an analysis of trends, levels and correlations. Ph.D. thesis, Demography and Sociology Program, Australian National University, Canberra

Hosseini-Chavoshi M, McDonald P, Abbasi-Shavazi MJ (2006) The Iranian Fertility Decline, 1981–1999: an application of the synthetic parity progression ratio method. Population 61(5–6):701–718

Kian-Thiebaut A (2002) Women and the making of civil society in post-Islamist Iran. In: Eric Hooglund (ed) Twenty years of Islamic Revolution: political and social transition in Iran since 1979. Syracuse University Press, Syracuse, New York, pp 56–73

McDonald P (2000) Gender equity in theories of fertility transition. Popul Dev Rev 26(3):427–440

Mir-Hosseini Z (2002) Religious modernists and the "women question". In: Eric Hooglund (ed) Twenty years of Islamic revolution: political and social transition in Iran since 1979. Syracuse University Press, New York, Syracuse, pp 74–95

Salehi-Isfahani Dj (2008) Growing up in Iran: Challenging times for the Revolution's Children. Brown J World Aff 15(1):63–74

Salehi-Isfahani Dj, Egel D (2007) Youth exclusion in Iran: the state of education, employment and family formation, Middle East Youth Initiative Working Paper. Wolfensohn Center for Development, Dubai School of Government

Shadi-Talab J (2005) Iranian women: rising expectations. Critique: Crit Middle East Stud 14(1):35–55

Index

The manufacturer's authorised representative in the EU is Springer Nature Customer Service Centre GmbH, Europaplatz 3, 69115 Heidelberg, Germany. If you have any concerns regarding our products, please contact ProductSafety@springernature.com

Printed and bound by CPI Group (UK) Ltd, Croydon, CR0 4YY
30/09/2026
02225449-0005